Inspiration * Motivation * Perspiration

The NEW Fast-Edge Home Fitness Plan

By

Award Winning Trainer Kory Angelin

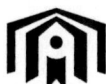

authorHOUSE™

1663 LIBERTY DRIVE, SUITE 200
BLOOMINGTON, INDIANA 47403
(800) 839-8640
WWW.AUTHORHOUSE.COM

First published by AuthorHouse 06/17/05

ISBN: 1-4208-5414-3 (sc)

Printed in the United States of America
Bloomington, Indiana

This book is printed on acid-free paper.

<u>ACKNOWLEDGE</u>

Thanks to Mom and Dad who have supported me my whole life and who I love very much. I appreciate the rest of my family too and could not have gotten where I am today without your support. Thank you to Dawn who gives me great inspiration and motivation everyday. Thanks to Scotty for stepping up to the plate when no one else would. To Jay, great pictures.

PREFACE

I am writing this book for the millions of people who choose not to exercise and eat right. Can anyone walk into a bookstore anymore without being hand fed diet books such as "The Zone", or "The South Beach Diet"? My intentions, therefore, are to bring about a fundamental approach to not only eating healthier but developing an exercise program as well, all from the comforts of home.

As a former college athlete and competitive bodybuilder now, I know the hardships of sound nutrition and self-motivating exercise. For my latest bodybuilding competition, I had lost thirty-seven pounds in just ten weeks. It was a daunting and grueling task but one that is necessary to excel in the sport. It requires a multitude of increasing and decreasing the amount of daily calories. Although extreme, an effective nutrition and exercise program can help in achieving any goal one might have. For me, it was about discipline since I needed to lose thirty-seven pounds to compete. This level of activity, in my early years, led me to my chosen career path. I hold a degree in Sports Medicine, as well as, am certified as an Athletic Trainer, Fitness Instructor, and Specialist in Performance Nutrition.

Upon seeing how little the average person exercises and how their nutritional programs equal that of your average pig, I decided to start my own business called FAST-EDGE. For the last seven years, my company has trained thousands of high school, college, and professional athletes. The type of training, however, is not your typical regimen of weight training. It consists more of a circuit geared toward speed, strength, and agility drills.

We couple that with a sound nutritional program based on individual needs and we produce some of the best athletes in America. Since our circuit training produced remarkable results, I took that concept and applied it to the average person who rarely exercises. I wanted to combine the elements of nutrition and training of our athletes and gear it for the person looking to shed a few pounds. Since the average cost of a gym membership is over $400 dollars per year, the goal was then to apply that circuit method for ones home. This home exercise plan will then prove that it does not take a health club to make you health-y.

The design of this book is not intended to be overly scientific. This book is a straight forward nutritional and exercise plan to make the average person healthier, all from the comforts of home. You will learn how to make a gradual change in lifestyle rather than a drastic one. This gradual change will prove to be the key to success.

TABLE OF CONTENTS

APPENDIX I
GLYCEMIC INDEX OF COMMON FOODS*
93

APPENDIX II
VITAMINS
94

CHAPTER ONE
LET'S GET MOTIVATED

What is it that gets you up in the morning? What is it that enables you to go into work five days a week, month after month, year after year? What is it that helps to push out those last couple of reps at the gym? The real question is **WHAT GETS YOU MOTIVATED?**

I truly believe that God gave me the gift to help motivate people to have a happy and healthier lifestyle. Before one takes a trip on this journey, they must understand that motivation plays a significant role for not only a sound body but a sound mind as well. One of the most productive ways to harness this motivation is by establishing a goal. I was fortunate enough to learn this from a very young age.

I grew up in a pleasant suburban town on Long Island. Growing up the youngest, two sisters and one brother, fed into my development of being competitive. Trying to out do one another was always a common theme around my house. If my sister had received a B on a test, then I would have to get an A. If my brother scored a touchdown in a football game, then I would have to score two. I was never one to settle for second best. My earliest recollections of self-motivation through goal setting occurred back in elementary school. I was eleven years old when it was time to partake in the always-cruel West Point Fitness Routine. You see this was not your ordinary day in gym class where one shared a friendly game of badminton. This event took place once a year and assured me its sole existence was there only to separate the "boys" from the "not so boys". The test consisted of a variety of agility and strength moves such as jumping, cutting, balancing, and the always feared- the pull up. You see the pull up was my one weakness- it was my kryptonite. Like any superhero, however, I set out to conquer this evil. My power breakfast that morning to get ready for the big event consisted of a healthy serving of fruity pebbles and two cookies. It was definitely one of the most nutritional meals of the day, or so I thought. As I made my way to the bus stop there was a great level of anxiety as each student was contemplating his or her own fate for the test. That morning lasted forever as we awaited our inevitable walk to gym class. There I found myself, third in line and in back of Johnny Smith, the best athlete in school. Johnny ran like a deer, jumped like a kangaroo, and can zip through this test as if he was Bruce Jenner. Upon seeing some of my fellow classmates achieve three, four, and even five pull-ups fairly easily, my trepidation started to subside. "How difficult could this be", I remember clamoring to myself. As I glanced out of the corner of my eye, Johnny had completed six pull-ups and established the school record. I was about to find out my own fate. The first event was the pommel horse, where one was supposed to leap over an enormous mass of rubber. Although I did not stick the landing, my leap was worthy of an Olympic gold. Following the pommel horse was the balance beam. The object of this beam was to walk to the other side without falling into the pit of lava or so I envisioned. That skill was done to perfection, leaving me with my Lex Luther of sorts-"the pull up". Although nervous, my confidence level was soaring. As I proceeded to grip the bar, my blood was pulsating throughout both arms. With every ounce that was left in my eleven-year-old body, I started to pull as hard as I could. To my dismay, however, I was unable to even get one. The shrieking sound of laughter came next which could only be coming from my fellow classmates. This turn of events caused an indescribable feeling in the pit of my stomach, which I vowed would never happen again. That was a defining day for me because I remember setting my first goal-one pull up.

There was just one year until the next West Point Fitness Test and I was motivated to achieve my goal of one pull up. Since I was only eleven years old, I did not posses a great deal of knowledge about strength training. My brother at the time, who excelled in high school football, had built a home gym in our basement. This would be the foundation for my next year of training. I practiced and trained throughout the next year in the hopes of conquering my performance of the past. As the day drew near my confidence level grew even stronger. Finally, the day of the West Point Fitness Test and the start of a new and improved me. Staring at the pommel horse, the first event, I rubbed the bottom of my Nike sneakers on the ground like that of a bull in a fight. I leaped over the horse like Paul Hamm, winking at the judges as I stuck the landing. I then sauntered over the balance beam as if it was ten feet wide. Finally, the pull up bar was waiting. "We meet again", I declared to myself and then grabbed on without hesitation. I pulled up once, then twice, and before you knew it I had achieved seven pull ups surpassing the great Johnny Smith to establish the school record. Achieving this great accomplishment in my life was a tremendous influence in choosing my future career path.

Many years later I had received my Sports Medicine Degree and set out to conquer the world. It was during these years that I really understood how unhealthy society really was. At twenty-two years old, I had taken my first job with a local Physical Therapy Clinic on Long Island. To my surprise, 80% of the people we treated were over seventy years old, certainly not what I had expected to be working with. These people were not only elderly and out of shape but they lacked the motivation to do something about it. We treated everything from simple ankle sprains to more debilitating conditions such as strokes. They all, however, had one thing in common and that was that exercise was the only way to improve their condition. Since I had always envisioned working with more of the active population, this lifestyle was slowly starting to take a toll on me. It was at this time when I decided to form my own company called FAST-EDGE. This company was going to be geared more for athletes to try to improve their conditioning level. It would focus on circuits of speed, strength, and agility exercises, which were a serious departure from teaching elderly people how to walk again. I proceeded to attend many seminars to understand the science behind what makes an athlete excel over the average person. What made an athlete fast and quick was determined by how explosive their legs were. After understanding the physiology why athletes excel, I developed a series of circuits to institute to them. These circuit programs will later become the foundation for our home exercise plan.

The difference of ability between an athlete and that of the average person is incredible. What separates them apart from each other is an athletes overwhelming motivation and drive to succeed. This is the primary reason why goal setting is so important. Your own personal goal, whether it's to score four touchdowns or to lose four pounds, must be set so that motivation can be generated from it.

A major factor to consider when setting your goal is to make sure that it is realistic or attainable. I once trained a thirty-five year old woman who was interested in getting back into the modeling world. After having a successful career in her early twenty's, she felt that she could have the same success now. At 5'8 and only 110 pounds, her goal was to lose ten pounds. Very often in this business you will find yourself playing psychologist rather than trainer and this situation was no different. How was I going convince this person that her initial goal was just unrealistic? Needless to say, after eight weeks of circuit training and five pounds lighter, she looked fantastic. One must learn that to be successful at a nutrition and exercise plan, attainable goals must be set. For most of America, that might simply mean to just start exercising in the first place. Since only 1% of America exercises, that leaves 99% without the motivation or knowledge to do it. For others, however, more attainable goals might include dropping one pound a week or one clothing size in a month.

The second big step once your goal has been set is to involve family and/or friends. Try to identify whom your closest family/friend is that you would like to confide in. This person should be someone who will pick you up when you are falling into despair. And make no mistake about it, you will experience some lows throughout the process. Explain to them what your goals are and that you would like them to be there as a source of inspiration and motivation from time to time. Do not underestimate the power and influence that your family/friends might have in achieving your own goal. I like to call this "The Buddy System". You would be surprised how many of my clients "buddies" have started their own exercise plan due to the encouragement they had given to others.

Whether you are heading to the Olympics or heading home to cook dinner for the family, these two steps will help as motivational tools for success. There are, however, some other contributing factors to help motivate you to start or continue an exercise and nutrition plan. You should really pay attention to these next five words- **GET RID OF YOUR SCALE!** Unless you are planning on using it as a decorative plant stand, throw the scale in the garbage. This has been proven to be one of the single most contributors to frustration, and as we all know, frustration could deter ones motivation. If it is one aspect I have learned from the last fifteen years in this business, it is to not pay attention to what a person weighs. It is imperative when you are setting your realistic goals to not concentrate on how many pounds on a scale to lose but rather how much body fat to decrease. As stated earlier, goals such as one to two pounds a week are realistic, whereas, ten is not. One of the biggest complaints I hear is "Why isn't the scale moving when all I have been doing is exercising and eating right"? The primary reason for this is because a person is made up of a percentage of lean muscle and a percentage of body fat. Someone who is obese has a higher percentage of body fat and a low percentage of lean muscle. Conversely, an athlete for example has a higher percentage of lean muscle and a low percentage of body fat. Taking this into consideration, when a person is losing fat, they are also increasing their lean muscle, thereby, keeping the total volume in the body approximately the same. The majority of the population, however, assumes that there will be a significant drop in the scale. Although this does occur, the results may not be so evident on a scale. What you are more likely to see over the long run is a change in how your clothes fit and how much body fat is lost (*see chart below*). By paying too much attention to results on a scale, you are setting yourself up for failure. Motivation will undoubtedly turn to frustration, which will eventually steer you in the wrong direction.

AVERAGE BODY FAT %

	MEN	WOMEN
VERY FIT	6-12%	13-17%
FIT	12-17%	17-22%
SLIGHTLY OVERWEIGHT	18-24%	23-26%
OBESE	25%+	27%+

*Adapted from the International Sports Science Association Manual.

Another source for motivation that often gets overlooked is a series of before and after photographs. You know what they say- "a picture is worth a thousand words". It is alarming as to how viewing a photograph can help to motivate a person. Hollywood helps to prove this theory as well. How else did Rocky defeat Ivan Drago in Rocky 4? As we all know it was the picture of

Ivan on the mirror that helped Rocky motivate himself to train. Although you are not training to defeat a mammoth Russian, a picture could prove useful. I would recommend taking an initial photograph in just shorts and/or bra. Use that as a motivational tool before you embark on your new fitness program. Target your weak areas and envision how you would like them to look. Every month thereafter snap another photograph of yourself and bask in the glory as you see yourself whither away to nothing. For my last bodybuilding competition that I competed in my goal was to weigh 163 pounds. This weight class would put me in the middleweight division where I was confident I could excel. I started out my program taking a picture of myself at which time my weight was 200 pounds. Since my goal was to lose approximately thirty-seven pounds, my initial picture was used as a motivational tool for success. Training two times a day, six days a week requires a tremendous amount of discipline and motivation. As the first month passed, I snapped my second photograph where, surprisingly, there was already a tremendous change from the previous one. This process was continued for the next three months where finally, my goal weight was achieved.

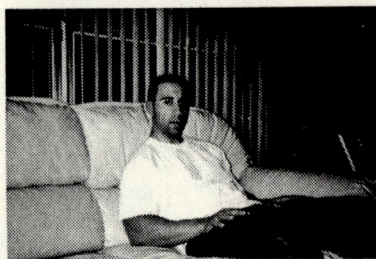 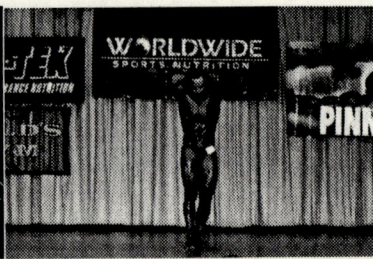

BEFORE AFTER

This next source of motivation could be a wake up call for some. I like to describe it as "The Scare Tactic". It is termed this because it uses fear as the overwhelming source for motivation. Let me explain: when I first started out many years ago as a trainer, I was contacted by a woman who was interested in starting a work out program. This woman, in her early forty's, had never exercised a day in her life and was a little apprehensive about starting. After taking her health history, however, I learned that both her parents and grandparents had a history of cardiovascular disease. It was this information that gave her the motivation and determination to start a program. She did not want to become a victim of her past. It, simply put, scared her. By acknowledging this information from the start, it was used in a positive way. Anyone starting out on an exercise and nutrition plan should inquire about his or her own health history. Most people I come in contact with could say that they know there is a history of cardiovascular disease but could not identify everyone who has had it. A person should always remember to have a yearly physical done to identify any change in cholesterol or blood pressure. If you are about to work with a personal trainer for the first time, he/she should conduct an initial health assessment. A good health assessment will include such tests as body fat percentage, activity level, blood pressure, heart rate, and health history to name a few.

I, personally, recommend this next method for creating motivation and that is- "The Workout Partner." There are not enough fingers on my hand to count the amount of times I had gotten through a workout due to the encouragement of my workout partner. There is nothing better than the sound of chaotic screaming as you try achieving a few extra repetitions on an exercise, or the phone call at six in the morning everyday to make sure you are ready to leave for the gym. Nothing could compensate for the amount of motivation that this generates. Unlike "The Buddy System", described earlier, this person is along side of you every step of the way. For me, the workout partner has been my number one source of motivation and I have made it of utmost importance when I train. They feel the same amount of nausea as you get one more squat in, producing the same river of sweat as you try to perceiver through one more set of crunches, and feel the same amount of jubilance as your bodies morph into that of Adonis. It makes exercise an extremely fun activity rather than that of a chore. I attribute my four months of training, previously mentioned, to my workout partner. My program consisted of forty minutes of cardio (treadmill or efx) at 5:30 a.m., along with weight training and cardio at night. This type of program is extremely fatiguing and taxing on the body. Factor in the fact that my total calories for the day went from 3500 to 1500 in the course of two months and you have the makings of a nervous breakdown. This is what makes your partner as valuable as your workouts themselves. Also remember that you must motivate your partner as much as they motivate you. I remember one time exercising with a friend of mine. He was very fit and, at one time, excelled at college football. We decided that since either of us trained with anyone that it might be a good idea to train together. Our first workout consisted of an overall upper body circuit that started with the bench press. I started off as the spotter or the guy who ends up helping the last couple of repetitions of the set. As he struggled toward the end of the set, I remember screaming to try to motivate him to achieve a couple more. "Great set," I exclaimed, and as I was perched to grab the bar for my set, I expected the same amount of motivation. Instead, as I struggled at the end of the set, my partner stood there as though he had taken a vow of silence. Needless to say, that was the first and last time we ever trained together again. There is no question that, if chosen correctly, the workout partner could be a never ending well of motivation for achieving any health goal.

Understand that there is no one magic tool for inspiring or motivating someone to exercise and eat correctly. What works for one particular individual might not work for another. Hopefully, some of these factors might help lead you down that path of wellness. The following is a review list of some of the factors discussed earlier.

FACTORS TO HELP MOTIVATE

1. Goal Setting

2. "The Buddy System"

3. Before/After Photographs

4. "The Scare Tactic"

5. "The Workout Partner"

CHAPTER TWO
<u>HURDLE THE EXCUSES</u>

What is it about society's affinity for giving excuses? Is it because we are afraid of not succeeding? Does not succeeding mean we automatically fail? One should always remember that every successful person in this world has experienced one or more failures at some point in their lives. Learning from our mistakes is an essential ingredient in building our character. **If you don't experience the lows, you won't appreciate the highs.** Working in this business for many years has taught me two valuable lessons. The first lesson is to understand that people create excuses for everything. The second lesson is to never take those excuses personally. If I had a dime for every time someone gave me an excuse as to why they can't exercise or eat healthy, I would be rich. Since only 1% of the population exercises, it left me asking myself "what's the other 99% doing." To answer that question I first had to identify some of the most popular excuses out there. I decided to survey one hundred people. This target group consisted of both men and women, ages twenty to seventy-five. Fifty percent of the people polled were currently enrolled in an exercise and nutrition plan. Since they were already engaged in a plan, the question asked to them was "what is your number one excuse to miss a day of exercise". The other fifty percent of the people polled did not partake in any kind of exercise or nutrition plan. The question that was posed to them was "why do you not partake in an exercise program". In this chapter we will breakdown the three most common excuses and some suggestions on how to hurdle them.

Take the following quiz and see how you rate:

1. Which is the most important to you?

a)	Job- 1 point
b)	Money- 2 points
c)	Family Health- 3 points

2. Do you have a family history of cardiovascular disease?

a)	No- 1 point
b)	Yes- 2 points

3. Do you consider yourself overweight?

a)	No- 1 point
b)	Yes- 2 points

4. How many times per week do you exercise?

a)	3 or more- 1 point
b)	2- 2 points
c)	0 or 1- 3 points

RESULTS:

If you scored an 8 or higher, there should be no excuse as to why you are not on an exercise and diet plan at least two times per week.

"I Have No Time To Exercise"

If God only gave twenty-five hours in a day instead of twenty-four, then everyone could use that extra hour to exercise. Of course that is not the case and despite what people may think, twenty-four hours is enough time to be healthy. During my survey, no time to exercise was the most common excuse given. Does this sound like you?

"There aren't enough hours in the day"
"I have to get my kids ready in the morning"
"I have to cook dinner for my family"
"I worked 14 hours today"

Let us be honest, these are valid excuses, occasionally, but not every time. One hundred and sixty-eight hours in a week is enough time to find at least two hours to be devoted toward an exercise plan. This is why our home circuit program, discussed later, will be of great importance. The greatest benefit to this plan is the fact that it can all be achieved from the comforts of your home. No matter how many hours of work you put in, creating time for your own health is essential for both mind and spirit. Since my own schedule requires at least a fifty-five hour workweek, I still find time to exercise. Let me show you what I mean. My day begins every day of the week at the same time- 5:00 a.m. Although I am not the happiest pea in the pod to be up that early, I do find time to cook six egg whites to get me going. I start training clients from 6:30 a.m. to 12:30 p.m. It is then off to the gym where the next hour and a half is devoted to my own exercise program. Lunch is squeezed in afterward, usually some chicken and brown rice with a protein shake. Since I am constantly eating throughout the day, my body is sustaining its energy level. The next several hours include personal training for various athletes, bringing my total workday to thirteen hours. By the time I arrive at home there is enough time to prepare some dinner before retiring to bed. This day is repeated Monday thru Friday all year round. What separates me from the person that claims they have no time to exercise is the fact that I **prioritize.** For you to be successful at time management, prioritization is the key ingredient. If you put a healthy lifestyle at the top of your importance list, it will be easier to find time to do it. Ask yourself, "Is living a long healthy life important to me". If the answer is no then you are not ready to make the commitment for this life changing experience. If the answer is yes, you simply need to find a way to fit it in to your schedule. The home circuit plan, described later, consists of a variety of twenty-minute exercise circuits to be done weekly. These twenty-minute circuits really are a small price to pay for a healthy living. Adding this one-hour per week will undoubtedly change your life. The first concept that you must understand is that it is never too late to start an exercise program. Some of my most committed clients are over the age of sixty-five. They understand that exercise will help combat a variety of aging conditions, such as, arthritis and degenerative disk disease. The second concept, without sounding like a family psychiatrist, is to understand that "you" do matter. Start putting yourself first for a change because you are important as well. Too many people spend more time taking care of others and forget to do the same for themselves.

Once you have learned to make an exercise program a priority in your life, find a way to **schedule** it into your day. This might mean certain sacrifices may occur as a result of scheduling time for this plan. This may include having to give up watching your favorite soap opera everyday or the first three innings of a baseball game that is on. If these are ultimately so important that death would occur by missing them, then you might choose to wake up an hour earlier to start the program. Whichever the case, respecting that time devoted for exercise is essential. Do not have the attitude of "I will do it at some point today". Too many problems could arise from this scenario. The time is there, you just need to find it. This was never more evident than with a former client of mine. This particular female was forty years old and was married with two children, ages six and eight. In addition, she was also the Vice-President of a successful finance company where working fifty to sixty hours a week was a common practice. I typically trained her and her husband at their home three times a week. Since time was always an issue with her they had a gym constructed in their home. She would be so exhausted from working and taking care of the children that exercise no longer became a priority. Furthermore, the times she was actually awake to train she had no energy. I decided to explain to her that exercising was obviously not a priority to her. "Why wouldn't you want to live a long and healthy life and watch your kids grow up", I explained to her. She finally realized that she was not only being selfish to herself but to her children as well. From that day forward she made being healthy a priority in her life. Her way of sacrificing was to stop work one hour earlier, three times per week. For her, this made all the difference in the world both physically and mentally. She has since been one of my most dedicated clients over the past ten years.

The final phase, once you have scheduled time into your day is to be **disciplined** about it. While scheduling a time to train two to three times per week might seem easy, actually sticking with it for months to come is another story. Why else do most New Years resolutions fail come February- no discipline? One of the biggest New Years resolutions year after year is to start an exercise and nutrition program. It is also, however, one of the most common resolutions that is broken. When discipline starts to fade, think back to why you made your plan a priority in the first place. Whether you just wanted to shed a few pounds or lower your cholesterol, rehashing those thoughts will help.

One of the most common reasons I found during my survey as to why people do not have time is because they are unorganized. In life, **organization** plays a critical role in structuring a day. Just take a look at some professions such as teaching, accounting, and financial managing and you will find that organization plays a significant role. This also rings very true with couples that have children. Attempting to organize a schedule for yourself is tough enough, let alone for one or more children. What seems to be a successful remedy for this is to purchase a calendar. Mark down the days that you plan to exercise in that week. Many of my own clients have benefited a great deal just by purchasing a two-dollar calendar. Some people need to visually see that time blocked out for it to be of some importance.

These same principles are also true when it comes to eating healthy. Having no time to eat healthy tends to be my favorite excuse. Let me explain in the simplest of terms: if you eat food everyday, which is undoubtedly the case, then there should be no reason why it shouldn't be somewhat healthy. Is there some shortage of healthy food that only I seem to be unaware of? Of course, when put in to those terms it sounds ridiculous. The biggest problem people have in their home is the presence of "junk" food. My survey revealed that the reason for this excessive "junk" food was because of the kids. If you have it, you will eat it. There have been many occasions when meeting my home clients for the first time that I will rummage through their pantry throwing out anything of poor value. Although shocking, it is an alarming reminder as to what steps need to be taken to be successful at a nutrition plan. Eating healthy, as with exercising also needs to be a priority. Once this is accomplished, you could focus on scheduling it into your day. Since completely changing your diet is too drastic, you will learn later how to ease the transition. The nutrition plan, discussed later, will provide you with a progression of days to eat healthy. People who decide to try a variety of diets find that their weight is always fluctuating. These are referred to as "Yo-Yo dieters". We will learn later why "Yo-Yo dieters" never succeed in achieving their goals. A gradual change as opposed to a drastic one will ensure success.

MAKE "NO TIME" INTO "GO TIME"

1. Prioritize

2. Schedule Time Into Day

3. Be Disciplined

4. Organization

"*I Am* ***Too Tired*** *To Exercise*"

Feeling too tired to exercise was the second most popular excuse given on my survey. I, personally, experience this excuse at least once a day with my own clients. There always seems to be the inevitable phone call at which point you hear the faint voice on the other end say, "I went to bed late and I'm just too tired to make it there". There have been multiple times where I have gone to the gym feeling exhausted and left feeling invigorated. People do not seem to realize that the more you exercise, the greater amount of endorphins is released in the body. It is this reaction that will help in giving you more energy throughout the day. Feeling 100% everyday of your life is just unrealistic. There are many factors that contribute to feeling tired. The most obvious one is lack of sleep. Lack of sleep tends to be the biggest contributor to feeling unenergetic. Doctors advocate that the average person should have at least eight hours of sleep a night. In a perfect world this might be true but as we all know that is not the case. People have responsibilities such as jobs and families to take care of. Living in this very stressful and fast paced society does not help with obtaining this many hours of rest. Using this as an excuse should only be warranted when you truly are exhausted. There must be a concerted effort to obtaining a peaceful nights rest.

There are some ways, however, to overcome this feeling. What tends to be successful for some people is to **establish a set time** or pattern to go to bed at night. Attempt to follow a routine throughout the week. It might include watching your favorite show at ten o'clock and then hitting the sack or reading a chapter in a book before retiring to bed. The body, over time, will eventually adapt to that time or pattern enabling you to fall asleep faster. You would be surprised how many of my clients have benefited from this advice. Although it sounds very simple it is one of the best techniques in getting a good nights rest.

Another major contributing factor to a person's energy level is the intake of high glycemic carbohydrates. This has been the focus of many diets out today. Examples of this include white starchy foods such as pasta, breads, cereals and rice. High glycemic carbohydrates, discussed in more detail later, have two effects on the body. The first effect on the body is a sharp rise in blood sugar levels. The second response is a sharp rise in insulin levels. The problem occurs when this sharp rise turns into drastic fall. When eating a bowl of pasta for example, the body will spike up insulin and sugar levels leaving you with a boost of energy. A few hours later, however, you will experience a feeling of fatigue as the body sharply drops these two levels. Most people experience this feeling a few hours after lunchtime. Since most of society loves to eat these high glycemic carbohydrates for lunch, they will experience that lull in the day at about three or four o'clock. **Low glycemic carbohydrates** tend to be the better choice because of its moderate increase of insulin and sugar levels. These foods include whole-wheat pasta, sweet potatoes, lentils and kidney beans to name a few. This moderate rise throughout the day will sustain a person's energy level rather than decrease it.

The ingestion of too much caffeine can also alter sleep pattern, which could result in decreased energy levels. There has been an outpouring of studies within the past decade of the effects of caffeine. It stimulates the central nervous system, which could lead to better awareness and concentration. It also affects the adrenal gland by stimulating fatty acid release. It results in very much the same way as high glycemic carbohydrates. By this I mean there is a sharp jolt in energy followed by a period of fatigue a few hours later. A majority of today's population, more than 75%, consumes caffeine, making it one of the most widely used drugs in America. As with many drugs, caffeine creates both positive and negative effects. Amongst the positive effects is that it acts as a vasodilator in the body. A vasodilator increases the size of your blood vessels allowing an increase in circulation. As circulation increases, so does metabolism. The faster the metabolism, the greater amount of calories is burned. The best way to harness this effect is to have a small cup of black coffee about one hour before you work out. This may help you in sustaining your workout longer. Caffeine, however, turns negative four to five hours later when energy levels drop drastically- similar to that described earlier. Some people, in addition to drops in energy level, experience anxiety as a result of caffeine. Caffeinated drinks have always been widely used in society. Today, energy related drinks are amongst the most popular. With a greater number of people buying into energy drinks, an understanding of its effects should be known. **Decreasing the amount of caffeinated drinks** consumed could lead to a more sustained energy level. One of the first elements I look at with a client is what he/she drinks and at what time they are drinking it at. For example, if a person enjoys a cup of coffee after dinner, it might result in a restless nights sleep. The result will be felt the next day, however, when the effect of not sleeping begins. Caffeine is also present in foods containing chocolate. Many runners make it point to consume a candy bar of some kind to boost energy levels. In fact, it has become a common practice in many sports. The effects of chocolate though are similar to that of a cup of coffee. It seems harder, however, for society to give up their chocolate than it is to give up their coffee.

CAFFEINE CONTAINING FOOD/BEV.

Pepsi (1 can, 12 oz.)	**38 mg.**
Coke (1 can, 12 oz.)	**45 mg.**
Coffee (Reg., 8 oz.)	**130 mg.**
Coffee (Decaf. 8 oz.)	**3 mg.**
Chocolate Cake (1 slice)	**14 mg.**

The last factor, which could alter energy levels, is stress. What person does not experience stress on a daily basis? Whether it is job or family related, stress seems to be a popular reason why people feel run down. Although there is no definitive solution to decrease stress, one should start by identifying what it is that is causing it. Typically, worrying about money tends to be a popular answer. Stress is not only known to cause irregular sleeping patterns but is also linked to more serious conditions such as heart attacks. It certainly should not be taken lightly. Getting a **yearly physical** is a step in the right direction. It will provide you with important physical data such as cholesterol and blood pressure levels.

FEEL "WIRED", NOT "TIRED"

1. Establish Pattern For Sleeping

2. Decrease Amount Of High Glycemic Carbs.

3. Decrease Amount Of Caffeinated Food/Bev.

4. Obtain Yearly Physicals By Physicians

"I Am In Too Much Pain To Exercise"

The third top excuse given as part of my survey has to do with pain. No one actually enjoys pain; therefore, it becomes a popular excuse to give to get out of a training session. This usually applies to the individual that exercises sporadically. These people never give their body a chance to adapt to the physiological changes that take place as a result of exercise. Before I elaborate on that, let us take a look at the body's response to stimulus and how it creates both soreness and pain.

How many times have you heard it, "No pain, No gain"? Although this statement has some validity to it, it is not quite as simple as it sounds. The biggest misconception with people is the difference between muscle soreness and pain. There is a distinct difference between these two responses of the body. Exercising requires a muscle to experience a series of repeated contractions. These very same muscles rely on a sufficient amount of fuel (glycogen, free fatty acids) and oxygen. Activity without pain means that the oxygen used meets the oxygen demands of the activity. Conversely, when the oxygen demands exceed the oxygen used, a byproduct called lactic acid is released into that area. Most people describe this feeling as a "burning" sensation in the muscle. To feel this effect, try leaning up against a wall and then hold a squat for one minute. A burning sensation will start to occur in the thighs after about one minute. The body is starting to release lactic acid to the thighs because of the lack of oxygen. It is the next twenty-four to seventy-two hours where most people do not understand the effects of this. Lactic acid typically remains in the muscle for twenty-four to seventy-two hours post exercise. The basic response is to perceive this sensation as pain, when in fact you are experiencing muscle soreness. For example, pain would be experienced if you were to fracture a bone or sprain a ligament, where as, simple exercise would create more soreness in the muscle.

The next step is to try to relieve that discomfort so you are not afraid to workout again. The single biggest mistake people make when they feel soreness from exercise is to remain sedentary. The longer you remain inactive, the longer the lactic acid remains in the effected area. The best way to combat that soreness is to **be very active** throughout the day. I make it a point before every training session to explain to my client what he/she might feel the following day. If I am putting my client through an intense leg workout, for example, I would explain to them to walk on the treadmill the next day to flush the lactic acid out of that area. This way he/she is not in a state of shock when they feel some leg soreness.

Another great method to combat pain and soreness is to **stay hydrated**. How many times have you heard that? It is alarming as to how many people actually adhere to this advice. The more hydrated an individual is, the greater the likelihood of flushing the lactic acid out of the affected area. Staying hydrated is one of the most fundamental concepts when exercising but one of the least practiced. People who often complain of soreness and muscle spasm following a workout are often the least hydrated. According to the American College of Sports Medicine (ACSM), you should drink 400-600 ml of fluid about two hours before exercise to promote hydration. The larger the amount of fluid in your stomach, the faster it will replace the loss of fluids in the body. Water, as well as, a variety of sports drinks will aid in this process. The one benefit a sport drink has over water is the addition of carbohydrates, which will aid in energy.

NO PAIN, ALL GAIN

1. Remain Active

2. Stay Hydrated

CHAPTER THREE
NUTRITION 101

The point of this next chapter is not to confuse you like a college level nutrition course. It is, however, going to teach you some basic information about nutrition. For as long as I could remember being a fitness trainer, people still think that you could obtain six pack abs from just doing sit ups. In fact, I always make it a point to tell people that the key to losing body fat has more to do with your diet than it does your exercise program. It actually breaks down to about an 80/20 split- 80% nutrition, 20% exercise. It does not matter how many sit ups you do a day, if you are not eating well, your body fat will continue to cover your muscle. Many nutritional books that I come across seem far to advanced for the average reader. In this chapter we will learn about carbohydrates, protein, fats and what they all do to the human body. Studies done over the past twenty years have concluded that a healthy nutrition plan will increase a person's daily performance. Let us first look at the basics.

Nutrients are an essential ingredient for the body to function. Most nutrients are classified into either Macro or Micronutrients.

MACRONUTRIENTS:

Macronutrients are a daily requirement of the body and are needed in large amounts. They are important in providing the body with energy, growth and repair. Carbohydrates, Protein, Fat and Water are all classified as macronutrients.

CARBOHYDRATES

According to the International Sports Science Association (ISSA), the average daily intake of carbohydrates is 287 g. for adult males and 177 g. for adult females (1 gram of Carbs. = 4 kcal.). At least 50% of your total calories for the day should be derived from carbohydrates. This percentage will typically be higher for athletes and people with a higher activity level. I can't tell you how many people gasp when I tell them that 50% of what you eat should be carbohydrates. We will learn, however, the difference between "good" and "bad" carbohydrates. There was once a day when carbohydrates were thought of as the anti-Christ. Of course, now, we know that not to be the case. In fact, they play a major role for the human body. There are so many misconceptions about this macronutrient that it is important to understand some basic functions of them.

Carbohydrates main function is to provide the body with its primary source of energy. When an individual exercises, for example, the first substance that is burned for energy is carbohydrates. It is also, however, the most abused nutrient. This has led to the rising level of obesity in America today. Many fast-food chains have recognized this and have introduced low carb. menus as a result. Once you understand the main function of carbohydrates, it is important to know that there are different types.

Carbohydrates fall into two main categories:
1) Simple
2) Complex

Simple Carbohydrates include molasses, honey, corn syrup and table sugar. They can also be present in dairy products as lactose and in fruit as fructose. They are referred to as simple because they contain only one or two sugar molecules. Typically, diets high in simple carbohydrates do not benefit the body. Complex carbohydrates, on the other hand, include fiber and starch and are found in grains and potatoes to name a few. They are important because they provide minerals, vitamins and other nutrients that help to fight disease and infection. Starch is a major energy source for the body and is typically found in veggies, pasta, breads and grains. Therefore, when people say to decrease carbohydrate intake they are primarily talking about simple or "bad" carbs. People refuse to believe that there are "good" and "bad" carbohydrates. Without understanding this concept, it will make achieving results very hard.

When a food is consumed the body responds in two ways. The first response is a rise in blood sugar level and the second is a rise in insulin level. Any consumption of a high sugared or "bad" carbohydrate will result in a **rapid** rise in these two levels. This is usually associated with a feeling of fatigue. The insulin will then store glucose and eventually convert any excess to body fat. The other negative is that high sugared carbohydrates will leave you with an increased appetite and craving for more sugar. The goal then is to consume lower sugared or "good" carbohydrates, which will provide the body with a **steady** rise in sugar and insulin levels throughout the day. What are some "good" and "bad" carbohydrates? "Bad" carbohydrates consist of simple sugars and white-floured products such as pasta, breads, and cereals. "Good" carbohydrates on the other hand consist of wheat-based products such as wheat bread and wheat pasta. When a wheat starch is consumed, the body will respond by releasing glucose at a slow steady rate.

One of the best tools I recommend to people is the Glycemic Index Scale. Foods are rated as a percentage based on the effects it has on blood glucose levels. By consuming lower glycemic foods or "good" carbohydrates, you will maintain that steady rise in insulin and sugar levels discussed previously. By consuming higher glycemic foods or "bad" carbohydrates your glucose levels will rise more rapidly, resulting in a negative affect. A low glycemic Index food is generally 40% or lower, 41-70% is for moderate glycemic foods and 71-100% for high glycemic foods. Keep in mind that by cooking a food, its carbohydrate make up is altered. Every meal should consist of a carb., protein and fat. Eating a lower glycemic carbohydrate will lower food cravings. This concept is one of the most important to understand when trying to change your nutritional plan. It is also the basis for our meal plan discussed later. **(SEE APPENDIX I FOR G. I. SCALE)**

PROTEIN

As with carbohydrates, protein plays an essential role in the human body. A person's diet should consist of about 25-35% protein. The RDA recommends that protein for an adult should be .8g per kg. of body weight (2.2 kg=1 pound). Among proteins main functions are growth, repair and production of enzymes, hormones and DNA. In certain instances, however, it is sacrificed for energy usually due to malnutrition and exercise. A good example of this can be illustrated with breakfast. How many times have you heard the question, "what is the most important meal of the day?" Although most people say breakfast, they really do not understand why. As we have discussed earlier, the human body's primary choice for energy is carbohydrates. It is the first substance burned when energy is needed. What is important to note is that you have a ten-hour window to consume a carbohydrate before the body starts to burn its second choice- protein. This simply put means if you go more than ten hours without consuming a carbohydrate, the body will start to burn protein instead. The problem with this response is that protein is found in muscle and should not be broken down to be used for energy. In fact, muscle should be preserved at all times. Therefore, let's say you go to bed at ten o'clock and wake up at seven a.m.. That is already nine hours without eating a carbohydrate. Now, let's say you skip breakfast, which most people do any way, your ten hour window has passed and your body is now forced to burn protein. This is what makes having a balanced breakfast so important. The goal should always be to have an adequate supply of protein to preserve lean body mass.

Proteins also act as antibodies, which the immune system creates when an infection is present. Therefore, it plays a huge role in disease prevention. The body's immune system, however, becomes weak when there is an insufficient amount of protein present in the body.

Proteins are actually made up of amino acids, which are used to spare muscle breakdown during activity. Without these amino acids, proteins could not be formed. This is typically the reason why amino acids are referred to as "the building blocks" of protein.

There are two main categories of amino acids:
1) Essential
2) Non-Essential

Essential

There are about nine essential amino acids. They are essential for the human body and are derived from the food we eat. The following is a list of the nine essential amino acids:

ESSENTIAL AMINO ACIDS	
VALINE	LYSINE
THREONINE	ISOLEUCINE
LEUCINE	HISTIDINE
PHENYLALANINE	
METHIONINE	
TRYPTOPHAN	

Non-Essential

There are eleven non-essential amino acids. They are also required for life but are not available through what we eat. Instead, they are manufactured within the human body. The following is a list of the eleven non-essential amino acids:

NON-ESSENTIAL AMINO ACIDS	
TYROSINE	GLYCINE
ALANINE	CITRULLINE
SERINE	PROLINE
ORNITHINE	CYSTINE
GLUTAMIC ACID	ASPARTIC ACID
AGANINE	PROLINE

Although cooking denatures or chemically alters an amino acid or protein, most are digested efficiently by the body. Animal meat tends to be the most efficient, while proteins from cereals, veggies and fruits are slower to be absorbed. In general, protein is found in poultry, meat, fish, eggs, milk, cheese, yogurt and soy based products. It is important to note that too much protein can lead to fat production. When protein is consumed, the body only uses what it needs for a specific function. If there is an excess present, the body will use it as either energy or store it as body fat. This is one reason why high protein diets are dangerous. Specifically, an increased consumption of animal meat can lead to a rise in cholesterol, due to the increase in saturated fat. Excess is also detrimental to the kidneys. When proteins are broken down they produce toxins in the body. These toxins are then sent to the kidneys to be filtered, however, overworking them in the process.

NITROGEN BALANCE

Nitrogen, which only proteins contain, can be useful in determining a person's protein requirement. The amount of dietary nitrogen ingested should equal the nitrogen excreted. Nitrogen is usually lost either through the skin when sweating or excreted through stool and urine. If you were to increase lean muscle through exercise, you would be in positive nitrogen balance. Conversely, if the body were tearing down muscle tissue to be used for energy, you would be in negative nitrogen balance. This phenomenon is especially important for athletes. Athletes always tend to want to increase their muscle mass, which is the reason why they should always be in a positive nitrogen state.

FAT

Lipids make up the third major macronutrient. Fats are primarily found in meats, fish and plants. Although it may be difficult to understand, every meal should contain a fat. This is not a misprint because fat plays a major role in the body. Among them are to provide insulation; contain essential fatty acids which help to maintain integrity of cell membranes; help to absorb fat soluble vitamins such as A, D, E and K; and serve as a source of energy. Too much, however, of the wrong kind of fats can lead to many diseases such as obesity, coronary heart disease, and high cholesterol. 15-20% of your total caloric intake should be derived from fats (1 g=9 kcal.). The average Americans diet, however, consists of about 40-50% fat, which explains the high level of obesity.

As with carbohydrates, there are also "good" and "bad" fats. Two of the most popular bad fats include saturated fats and cholesterol. A diet high in saturated fats and cholesterol has been proven to cause conditions such as heart disease and obesity. Fats can be categorized in three ways: Saturated, Polyunsaturated, and Monounsaturated:

SATURATED:

These fats are solid at room temperature and are commonly referred to as "bad" fats. They are found in hydrogenated vegetable products and most animal meat. This type of fat is not desirable to have in the diet because it prevents the flow of nutrients and oxygen throughout the body. Most people I come in contact with have a diet high in saturated fats.

MOST COMMON SATURATED FATS

HOT DOGS	PORK
BEEF	EGG YOLKS
MILK	BUTTER
CHEESE	CHOCOLATE
CREAM	SHELLFISH

POLYUNSATURATED:

These fatty acids tend to be liquid at room temperature. They are found in oils such as corn, soybean, sesame and sunflower. Since they are not solid they help to lower both HDL or "good" cholesterol and LDL or "bad" cholesterol. The one negative effect is that it will also lower HDL even if it is at a normal level. Omega 3/Omega 6 are two special types of polyunsaturated fats. They are termed fatty acids because the body cannot synthesize them. Omega 3's are among the best fats and are found in cold-water fish such as tuna and salmon, flaxseeds, walnuts and canola oil. They help in blood clotting; regulating blood pressure; and help to decrease risk of heart disease, stroke and cancer. Omega 6 fatty acids are found in animal and vegetable products like safflower and corn oils. They are important for growth and maintenance of the immune system but are a less desirable choice because they increase the risk for heart disease.

MOST COMMON POLYUNSATURATED FATS

PECANS	FISH
SAFFLOWER OIL	SOYBEAN OIL
ALMONDS	SUNFLOWER OIL
CORN OIL	

MONOUNSATURATED:

These fats are found in olive oil, canola oil and peanut oil. They affect the body by lowering just the LDL or "bad" cholesterol and increase the HDL or "good" cholesterol. Since cooking oil is a combination of all three, it is healthier to choose one with a high percentage of monounsaturated. Below is some popular cooking oils and their percent of monounsaturated fat:

OIL	%
OLIVE	75
CANOLA	55
CORN	20
COCONUT	10

As you could see, olive oil is among the best when cooking because of the high percentage of monounsaturated fat it contains. Conversely, corn is among the worst due to its low percentage of monounsaturated fat. The goal for everyone should be to maximize the intake of essential fatty acids and omega 3 and limit saturated fats and cholesterol. When exercising, the body will burn both carbohydrates and fats at an even rate. The longer, however, the exercise is prolonged, the more likely the body will burn fat. This is always the primary reason why experts say to perform a cardiovascular exercise for at least twenty minutes.

MOST COMMON MONOUNSATURATED FAT

PEANUTS	PEANUT BUTTER
PEANUT OIL	SESAME SEEDS
ALMONDS	AVACADOS
CASHEWS	CANOLA OIL
OLIVE OIL	

WATER

Water makes up the final macronutrient. It also remains as one of the most overlooked nutrients. Most people consume less than 8 oz. of water per day. The importance for staying hydrated is crucial for normal activity. Water helps to transport various chemicals throughout the body. Studies show that even a 4% drop in body water can have adverse affects in performance. Water can be typically lost through the skin by sweating; the mouth from exhaling; kidneys and feces. It is recommended for the average person to consume 8-12 oz a day. The general saying is that if you're thirsty, you are already dehydrated.

MICRONUTRIENTS

Although we tend to think of macronutrients first, micronutrients are also important. Micronutrients are otherwise known as vitamins and minerals. They serve many functions in the body. They aid in fighting infection by producing antibodies; help with proper nervous system function; and help in enzyme reactions. The following is a brief description of the vitamins and minerals and basic functions and examples of each. **(SEE APPENDIX II)**

CHAPTER FOUR
<u>FORGET ABOUT THE "FAD"</u>

Most people in today's society look for the fastest and easiest ways to lose weight. This is one of the reasons why there are so many "fad" diets out on the market today. If you don't believe me, take a ride to your local bookstore and marvel at the hundreds of diet books on the stands. Most of them claim to shed pounds fast and easy. Before we take a glance at some popular "fad" diets it is important to understand that there is no magic pill. You cannot just magically wake up one day and lose twenty pounds. Despite having a degree in Sports Medicine and Certification in Nutrition, almost everything I have learned has come from experience. Once you understand that every meal should consist of a carbohydrate, protein, and fat, you will be able to see the problems that arise with some diets. It is also important to note that not all diets are bad for you. The problem that I personally have is that most diets ask you to drastically change your lifestyle. There is a reason why most people on diets tend to put the weight back on after losing it initially. A drastic change in lifestyle will more than likely have a negative affect in the long run. The same principles apply when starting an exercise program. Instead of starting out with an advanced program, you should ease into a moderate workout plan so your body has time to adapt to it. Every one of my clients who have been on diets have all gradually gained the weight back. A gradual change, like you will learn in the next chapter, will give you better odds for succeeding. This will be the primary foundation for our nutrition plan discussed in the next chapter.

Let us take a brief look at some typical diets and how they claim to work:

"QUICK FIX"

Almost everyone has experienced this diet in some way. Two weeks until vacation and you are severely cutting back calories for fear of not fitting into your bathing suit. This is the underlying theory behind this type of diet plan. It is all based on severe calorie reduction. Although by cutting calories you will see a weight loss, it is extremely hard to stay on that path for the rest of your life. Remember, there is no magic pill.

EX: Cabbage Soup Diet, 5-Day Miracle Diet

LOW FAT/HIGH CARBOHYDRATE

The main principle behind this diet is to cut back on fats and increase carbohydrate consumption. By decreasing fat intake, you will virtually cut down on total calories consumed. Too much of a loss in fat, however, runs the risk of not getting enough essential fatty acids. As stated in the previous chapter, essential fatty acids help to decrease risk of cardiovascular disease. Since they also give a feeling of "fullness", severely decreasing them may lead to overeating in the long run.

EX: Hawaii Diet, Ornish Diet

CONTROLLING CARBOHYDRATE INTAKE

These include some of the most popular diets out today. The theory behind them is to stay on a firm proportion of carbohydrate, protein, and fat intake. The idea is to stabilize insulin and sugar levels in the body. Although reducing overall carbohydrate intake does produce weight loss it tends to be hard in the long run. As we have discussed earlier, carbohydrates are the body's first energy source. Although the body will burn fat in the absence of carbohydrates, it will compromise protein in the process. The "craving" for carbohydrates tends to be the downfall on these types of diets.

Other diets of this type recognize that "good" carbohydrates are essential. Some, however, advocate complete carbohydrate depletion for the first few weeks of the diet. This tends though to be unrealistic and too drastic. It is hard enough giving up carbohydrates for one day let alone a few weeks.

EX: Atkins Diet, South Beach Diet, Zone Diet

CENTERS FOR WEIGHT LOSS

This is one of the better choices because you are somewhat monitored. The problem, however, with some of these centers is that it focuses on weight too much. Many of them require weekly or monthly weigh-ins. My feeling is, as stated earlier, to throw away the scale and not worry about weight. The other negative factor is the cost. It is relatively expensive to join some of these centers. Factor in that they also require special food to be purchased and it makes it hard on the wallet.

EX: Weight Watchers, Jenny Craig

CHAPTER FIVE
FAST-EDGE NUTRITION PLAN

By now, you should have a good foundation for starting our nutrition and exercise plan. The problem with most diets, as stated earlier, is that they shock the body too fast. Remember, our programs intent is to provide a gradual change in lifestyle. The other positive aspect to our plan is that it will provide you with choices, which most diets do not provide. The plan will start in conjunction with the exercise program, which will be discussed in the next chapter. The goal, at first, will be to start on a two-day nutrition and exercise plan. Simply put, start out by setting aside two days a week for two weeks to eat right and exercise. After two weeks of getting comfortable with the plan, you will then add a third day of exercising and eating right. This will be followed for another two weeks until a fourth day is added. At this point in the program, you are working out and eating healthy four days a week. This should be the goal to achieve. If, however, you feel like you could add a fifth day of nutrition, there is a fifth meal plan included. There are five meal plans to be used as guides. Since every meal should include a low glycemic carbohydrate, protein, and monounsaturated fat, I have included three pages of each. This is where choices come into play. On this nutrition plan, you have the option to pick and choose whatever carbohydrates, proteins and fats you want. This way, you could formulate your own healthy meals. At every meal, just pick one low glycemic carbohydrate, protein and fat from their respective lists. This will ensure that the diet does not get boring.

The following is a list of "good" carbohydrates, proteins, and fats:

(1)
LOW GLYCEMIC CARBOHYDRATES

BREADS	CAL.
Whole wheat bread, 100% stone ground (1 slice)	60
Whole grain bread, (1 slice)	65
7 Grain (1 slice)	65
Whole wheat pita (1)	170
Oatmeal bread (1 slice)	73
Oats, cooked, (1 oz.)	100

CEREALS	
All bran (1/2 cup)	81
Raisin bran (1 cup)	190
Oat bran (1 cup)	120

PASTA/GRAIN/VEG.	
Whole wheat pasta (1 cup)	174
Lentils (1 cup)	230
Kidney beans (1 cup)	220
Chic peas (1 cup)	260
Sweet potato (1)	115
Spinach (1/2 cup)	20
Asparagus (1/2 cup)	20
Green beans (1/2 cup)	20
Squash, acorn, (1/2 cup)	60
Broccoli (1/2 cup)	22
Celery (1 stalk)	7
Cabbage, red/green, (1/2 cup)	9
Eggplant (1/2 cup)	13
Zucchini (1/2 cup)	15

DAIRY

Milk, 1%, (8 oz.)	100
Milk, fat-free, (8 oz.)	85
Cottage cheese, 1%, (1 cup)	160
Cottage cheese, reduced fat, (1 cup)	200
Yogurt, low fat, (8 oz.)	130
Yogurt, fat-free, (8 oz.)	127
Cheddar cheese, low fat, (8 oz.)	50

FRUIT

Apple, med. with skin	80
Cantaloupe (1 cup)	55
Grapefruit (1/2 cup)	40
Honeydew (1 cup)	60
Orange (1)	60
Pears (1)	100
Peaches (1)	35
Bananas (1)	103

(2)
<u>HIGH PROTEIN FOODS</u>

BEEF	<u>**CAL.**</u>
Flank (1 oz.)	50
Sirloin (1 oz.)	45
Buffalo burger (1 oz.)	30

POULTRY	
Chicken breast (1 oz.), no skin	30
Chicken breast (1 oz.), with skin	50

TURKEY	
Sliced (tyson), 3 slices	60
Light meat (1 oz.)	34

PORK	
Tenderloin (1 oz.)	35
Chops (1)	120

HAM	
Sliced (3 slices)	60

FISH	
Tuna steak (3 oz.)	150
Tuna canned (3 oz.)	110
Cod (3 oz.)	90
Flounder (3 oz.)	100
Salmon (3 oz.)	175

EGGS	
Whites (3)	56
Alternative, eggbeaters, (1/2 cup)	50

(3)
<u>FATS</u>

OILS/SPREADS	CAL.
Corn oil (1 tbspn.)	122
Canola oil (1 tbspn)	122
Olive oil (1 tbspn)	122
Margarine, soft, (1 tbspn)	40
Salad dressing, oil/vin., (1 tbspn)	45
Ketchup (1 tbspn)	15

(4)
DRINKS/SNACKS

DRINKS	CAL.
Water	0
Tomato juice (6 oz.)	30
Green tea (6 oz.)	3
Orange juice (8 oz.)	105
Apple juice	115
Grapefruit juice	85

SNACKS	
Almonds (3 tbspn)	160
Protein nutrition bar	200
Protein shake	200
Fruit (your choice)	

<u>MEAL PLAN 1 (1665 cal.)</u>
Weeks 1 and 2

Breakfast	Cal.
3 egg whites	56
½ cup cooked oats	148
Whole wheat bread (1 slice) w/jelly (preservative)	110
6 oz. grapefruit juice	170

SNACK	
1 apple	80
Water (8 oz.)	0

LUNCH	
Chicken breast (6 oz.)	180
Sweet pot. (1)	115
Iceberg lettuce (2 oz.)	8
Salad dressing, oil/vin., (1 tbspn)	45

SNACK	
Almonds (3 tbspn)	166
Protein shake	200

DINNER	
Beef, sirloin, (3 oz.)	135
Whole wheat pasta (1/2 cup)	87
Pasta sauce (2 oz.)	50
Apple juice (8 oz.)	115

MEAL PLAN 2 (1790 cal.)
Weeks 1 and 2

BREAKFAST	CAL.
Egg beaters (1/2 cup)	50
Raisin bran (1 cup)	190
Milk 1%, (8 oz.)	100
Whole wheat bread, 1 slice, w/jelly	110
Orange juice (8 oz.)	105

SNACK	
Pear (1)	100
Yogurt low fat, (8 oz.)	130

LUNCH	
Turkey (3 slices)	60
Whole wheat pita (1)	170
Cheddar cheese low fat, (1 oz.)	50
Iceberg lettuce (2 oz)	8
Salad dressing, oil/vin., (1 tbspn)	45
Green tea (6 oz.)	3

SNACK	
Protein bar (1)	200
Banana (1)	103

DINNER	
Pork chop	120
Whole wheat pasta (1 cup)	174
Pasta sauce (2 oz.)	50
Broccoli (1/2 cup)	22
Water	0

<u>MEAL PLAN 3 (1688 cal.)</u>
WEEKS 3 and 4

BREAKFAST	CAL.
Cottage cheese, reduced fat, (1 cup)	200
Oat bran cereal (1 cup)	120
Milk 1% (8 oz.)	100
Tomato juice (6 oz.)	30

SNACK	
Cantaloupe (1 cup)	55
Protein bar	200
Water (8 oz.)	0

LUNCH	
Buffalo burger (6 oz.)	180
Roll, whole wheat	75
Ketchup (1 tbspn.)	15
Green beans (1/2 cup)	20
Iceberg lettuce (2 oz.)	8
Salad dressing, oil/vin., (1 tbspn.)	45

SNACK	
Protein shake	200
Banana (1)	103

DINNER	
Flounder (6 oz.)	200
Sweet potato, w/skin	115
Broccoli (1/2 cup)	22
Water	0

MEAL PLAN 4 (2125 cal.)
WEEKS 5 and 6

BREAKFAST	**CAL.**
Egg whites (3)	56
Whole grain bread (2)	130
Jelly, strawberry preserve, (2 tbspn.)	100
Milk 1% (8 oz.)	100

SNACK	
Almonds (3 tbspn.)	160
Protein shake	200

LUNCH	
Chicken breast, no skin, (6 oz.)	180
Spinach (1 cup)	40
Pita, whole wheat	170
Pear	100
Apple juice (8 oz.)	115

SNACK	
Protein bar	200
Cottage cheese 1% (1 cup)	160

DINNER	
Steak, flank, (3 oz.)	150
Whole wheat pasta (1 cup)	174
Pasta sauce (2 oz.)	50
Asparagus (1 cup)	40
Water	0

OPTIONAL
MEAL PLAN 5 (1935 cal.)
WEEKS 7 and 8

BREAKFAST	**CAL.**
Waffle, oat bran, (2)	392
Pancake syrup, lite, (2 tbspn.)	50
Yogurt, low fat, (8 oz.)	130
Orange juice (8 oz.)	105

SNACK	
Apple	80
Cottage cheese 1% (1 cup)	160

LUNCH	
Turkey (6 slices)	120
Whole grain bread (2)	130
Cheddar cheese, low fat, (1 oz.)	50
Iceberg lettuce (2 oz.)	8
Salad dressing, oil/vin., (1 tbspn.)	45
Tomato juice (6 oz.)	30

SNACK	
Protein shake	200
Honeydew (1 cup)	60

DINNER	
Steak, sirloin, (3 oz.)	135
Kidney beans (1 cup)	220
Spinach (1/2 cup)	20
Water	0

CHAPTER SIX
FAST-EDGE FITNESS PLAN

ESSENTIAL EQUIPMENT

PHYSIOBALL: (med. size)

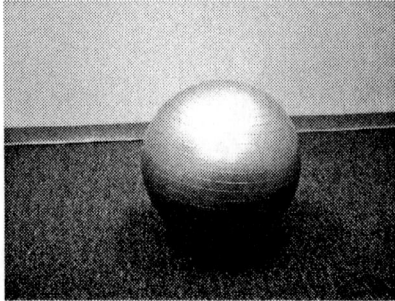

DUMBELLS: (1, 3, 5 pounds)

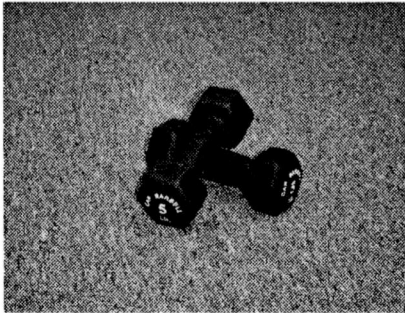

ANKLE WEIGHTS: (1-5 pounds)

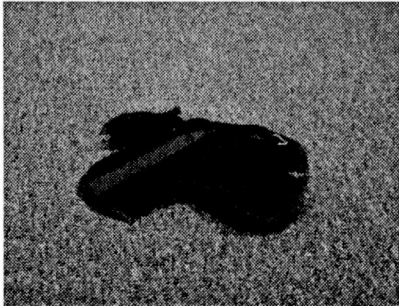

The goal of any weight training program is to increase lean and decrease body fat.

MYTH:
Lifting weights will make me too bulky.

FACT:
Lifting weights will make you too bulky ONLY if testosterone levels are extremely high and weight that is lifted is extremely heavy.

The FAST-EDGE Fitness Plan is designed to work out the entire body all from the comforts of home. The following are some reasons why I chose to develop a home fitness plan:

1) Less intimidating
2) Saves time
3) Free membership
4) Can be done at any time.

As stated earlier, these workouts are to be done in conjunction with the nutrition plans given in the previous chapter. The first two weeks consist of two days of eating healthy (meal plans 1 and 2), as well as, performing workouts 1 and 2 on those same days. Remember, the goal is to ease your way up to four workouts per week. There are both beginner and advanced programs for each work out. A person who is starting a workout program for the first time should follow the beginners program. Each program is designed as a circuit. A circuit is one of the most beneficial training methods used to create lean muscle and burn body fat. The idea is to keep the body moving so the heart rate remains somewhat elevated throughout the workout. The longer the heart rate is elevated, the more calories are likely to be burned. Therefore, our circuit consists of four exercises. Each exercise is performed for twenty seconds followed by twenty seconds of rest (20 sec. on, 20 sec. off). You are to move from one exercise to the next until all four exercises are completed. This will equal one successful circuit. Each workout will consist of performing eight circuits with a two min. rest period after the fourth circuit. The total workout time, therefore, is just twenty minutes. At the beginning of each program will be a review of exercises that will be used for that workout. If you feel like you need more rest time, then do not be afraid to take it. The goal is to accomplish eight circuits.

The following is a sample outline of what each workout will look like:

PRESTRETCH

EXERCISES 1-4: 20 SEC. ON, 20 SEC. REST
(Completion of all 4 exercises= 1 circuit)-perform 3 more times.

2 MIN. REST

EXERCISES 1-4 (same as above, 4 times)

POSTSTRETCH

PRE/POST STRETCHES

Each workout should begin and end with the following stretches. (5 sec. hold, 10x)

HAMSTRING STRETCH:
With 1 leg straight, slowly reach down toward foot with both hands (alternate legs).

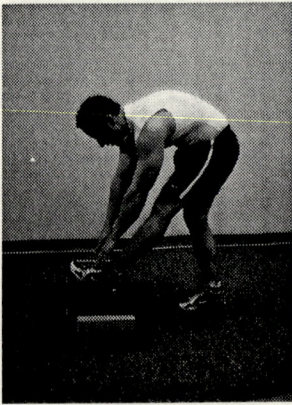

QUAD. STRETCH
Holding on to a stable surface with one hand, grab the opposite ankle until stretch is felt (alternate legs).

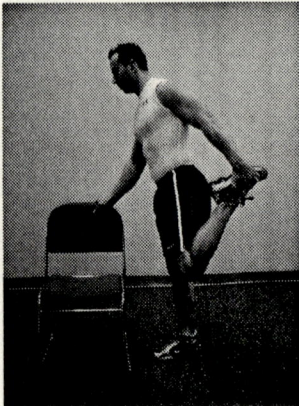

CALF STRETCH

On an elevated surface, slowly drop both heels toward floor until desired stretch is felt.

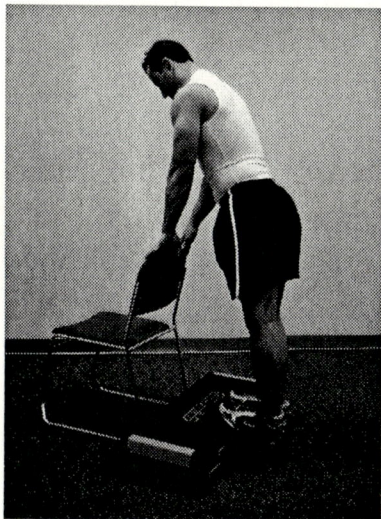

<u>PROGRAM 1 (REVIEW)</u>
(Squats, step-ups, push-ups, shoulder raises)

EXERCISE 1- BALL SQUATS
Target area- Legs

BEGGINNER: Start
Place ball on lower back. Feet are placed hip width apart. Keep feet far enough forward so when the squat is performed, the knees do not travel past feet. Hands remain on hips.

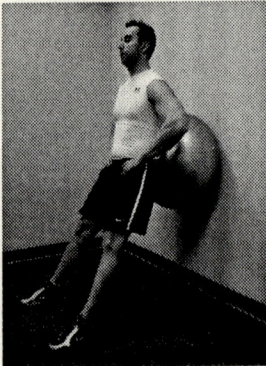

Finish:
Keeping the back straight, slowly drop butt toward floor until there is a 90-degree angle in knees.

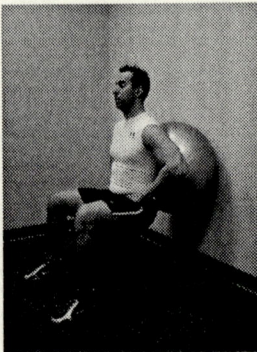

ADVANCED: Start

Place ball on lower back. Feet are placed hip width apart. Keep feet far enough forward so when the squat is performed, the knees do not travel past feet. Hold 5-pound dumbbells in each hand.

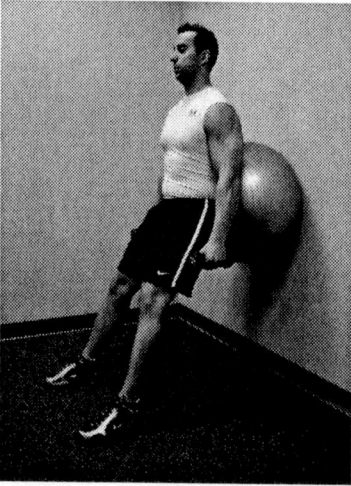

Finish:

Keeping the back straight, slowly drop butt toward floor until there is a 90-degree angle in knees.

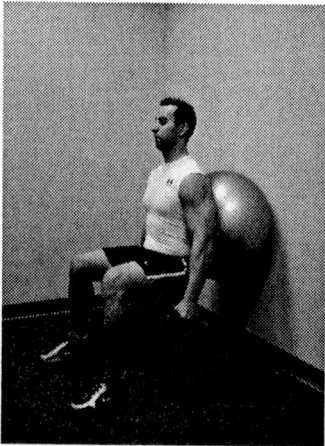

EXERCISE 2- **STEP-UPS**
Target area- Legs, cardio.

BEGINNER: Start
Find an elevated step in your house (ex: stairs). At a slow to moderate pace, step up onto the first step.

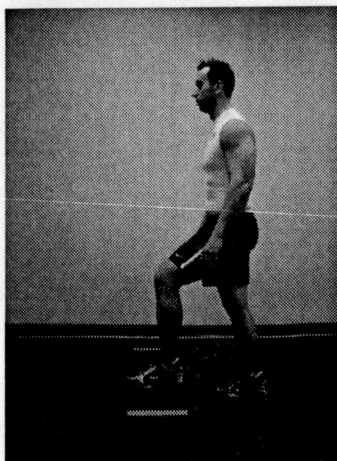

Finish:
Step down with same leg. Alternate leg every step.

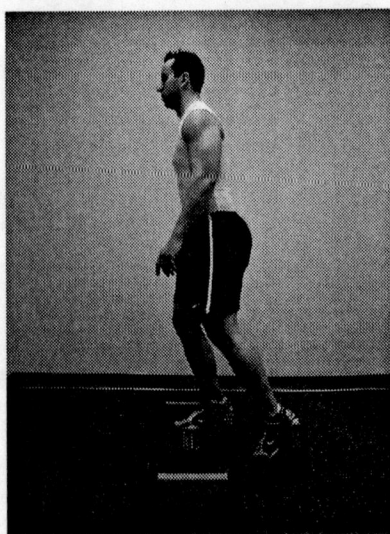

ADVANCED: Start

Place 5-pound ankle weights around each ankle. Find an elevated step in the house. At a fast rate, step up onto step.

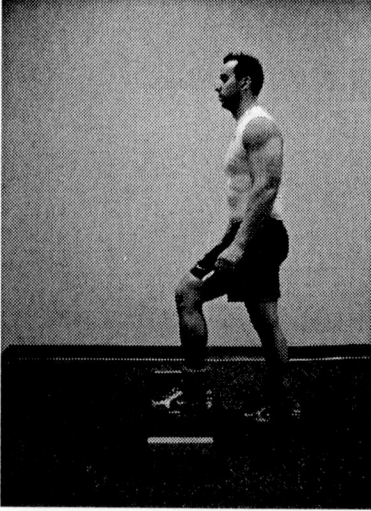

Finish:

Step down with same leg. Alternate leg every step.

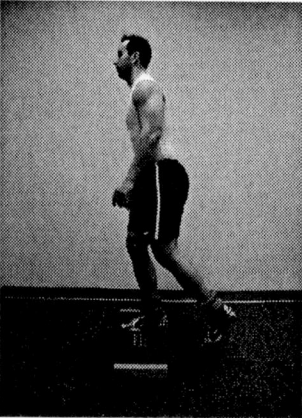

EXERCISE 3: **INCLINE PUSH UPS**

Target area- chest, shoulder, triceps

BEGINNER: Start

Find a stable countertop and place hands shoulder width apart. Place feet in back of you so your arms are taking on most of the weight. Slowly lower yourself toward countertop.

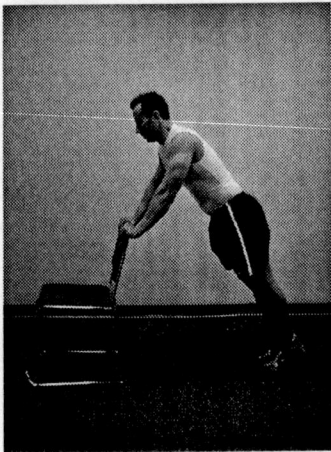

Finish:

Slowly push back up until arms are straight again.

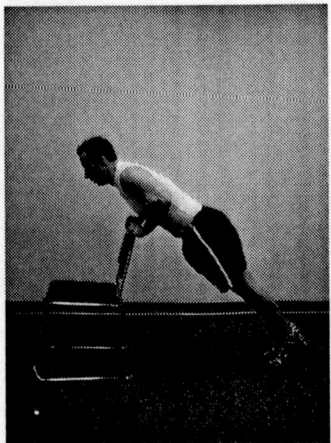

ADVANCED: Start

Find a stable countertop and place hands shoulder width apart. Place feet in back of you so your arms are taking on most of the weight. Slowly lower yourself toward countertop.

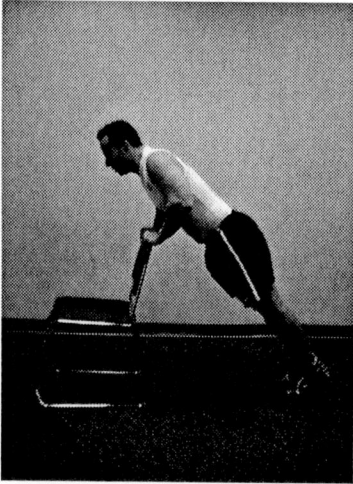

Finish:

Once you have reached the bottom, explode up so hands come off countertop. Relocate counter and start again.

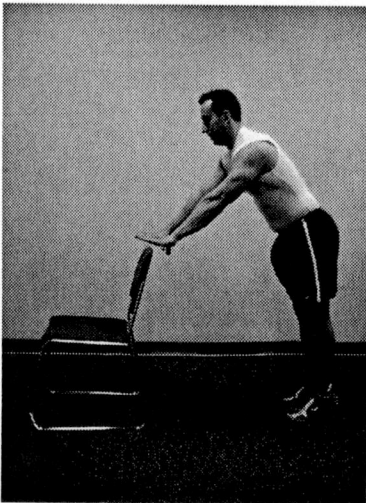

EXERCISE 4- **LATERAL SHOULDER RAISES**
Target area- Shoulders

BEGINNER: Start
Begin with feet hip width apart. Holding one-pound dumbbells, raise arms to side so they are parallel to ground. Keep elbows slightly flexed.

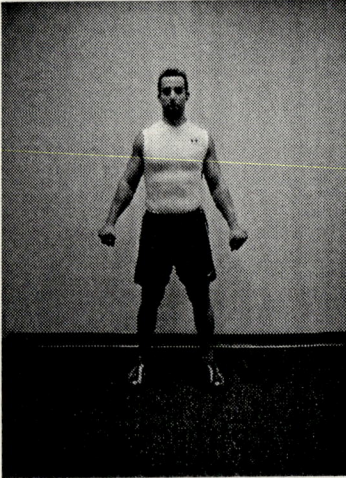

Finish:
Slowly lower both arms back to side.

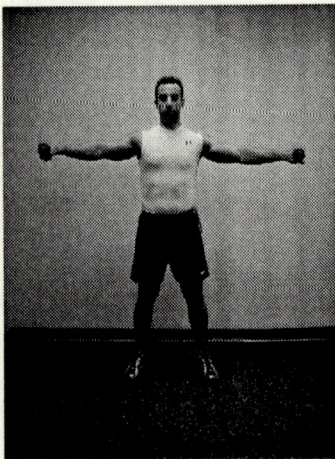

ADVANCED: Start

Sit on physioball with back straight, holding five-pound dumbbells. With elbows slightly flexed, lift arms out to side so they are parallel to ground.

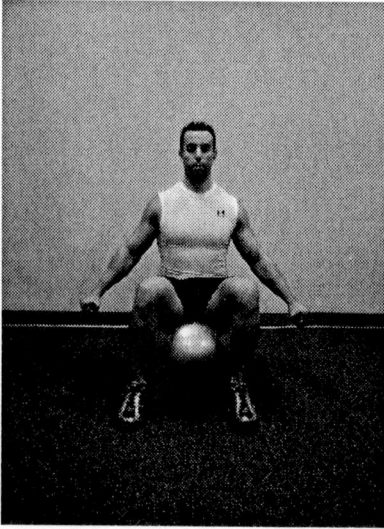

Finish:

Slowly lower arms back down.

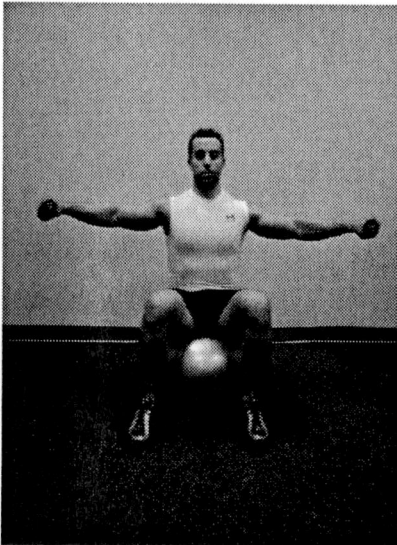

<u>PROGRAM 1 (WORKOUT)</u>
(Squats, Step-Ups, Push-Ups, Shoulder Raises)
WEEKS 1 and 2

PRESTRETCH

SQUATS- (20 sec. on, 20 sec. off)
STEP-UPS- (20 on, 20 off)
INCLINE PUSH-UPS- (20 on, 20 off)
SHOULDER RAISES- (20 on, 20 off)
Complete 4x total

2-MINUTE REST

SQUATS- (20 on, 20 off)
STEP-UPS- (20 on, 20 off)
INCLINE PUSH-UPS- (20 on, 20 off)
SHOULDER RAISES- (20 on, 20 off)
* Complete 4x again*

POSTSTRETCH

PROGRAM 2 (REVIEW)
(Squats, Shoulder Press, Step-Ups, Abs.)

EXERCISE 1- CHAIR SQUATS
Target area- Legs

BEGINNER: Start
Begin by sitting on the edge of a chair with feet hip width apart. Hold 5-pound dumbbells at side.

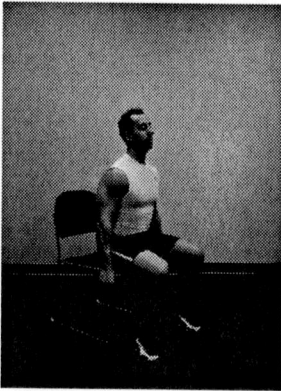

Finish:
Keeping the back straight, proceed to stand up.

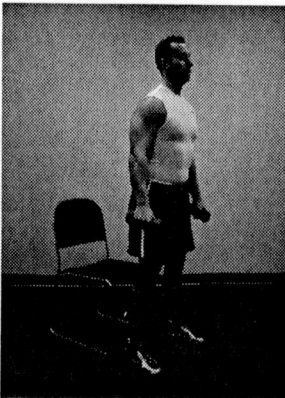

ADVANCED: Start

Sit on the edge of a chair with feet hip width apart. With the arms straight in front of you, hold a 5-pound dumbbell.

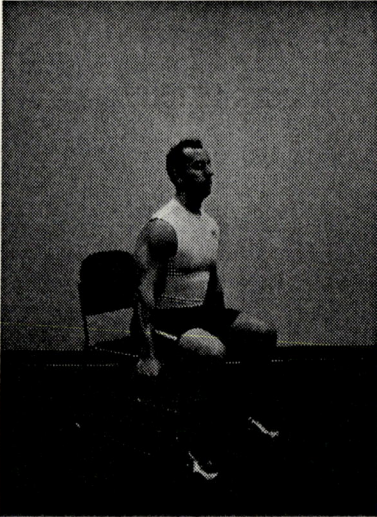

Finish:

Keeping the back straight, proceed to stand up. As you stand, lift arms until parallel to ground.

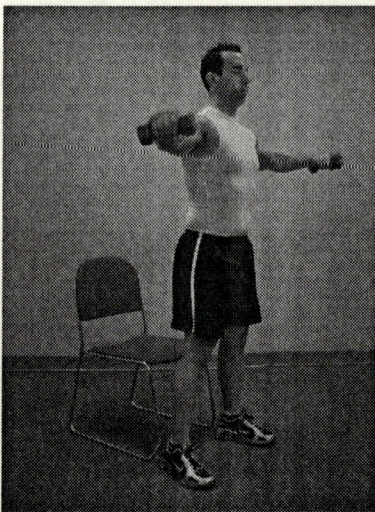

EXERCISE 2- **SHOULDER PRESS**
Target area- shoulders

BEGINNER: Start
Sit on the edge of a chair with feet hip width apart. Keep the back straight. Hold 3-pound dumbbells at side of your ears.

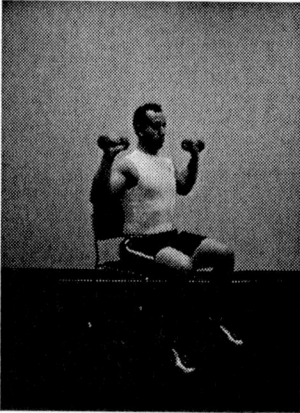

Finish:
Push dumbbells straight overhead, keeping the back straight.

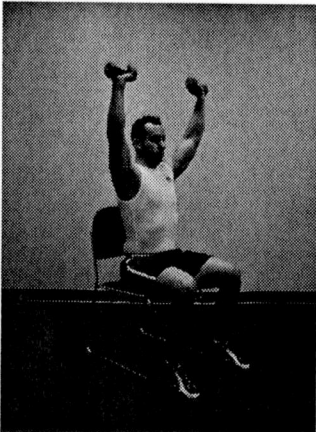

ADVANCED: Start
Sit on physioball with the back straight. Hold 5-pound dumbbells at side of ears.

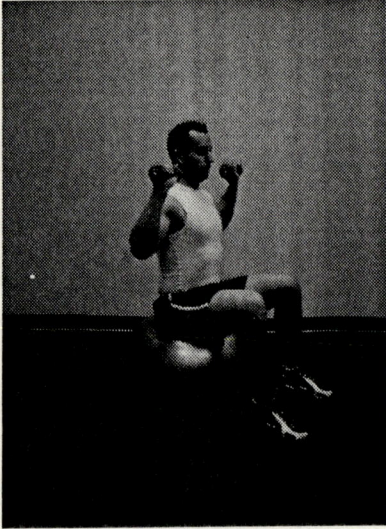

Finish:
Keeping the back straight, push arms straight above head.

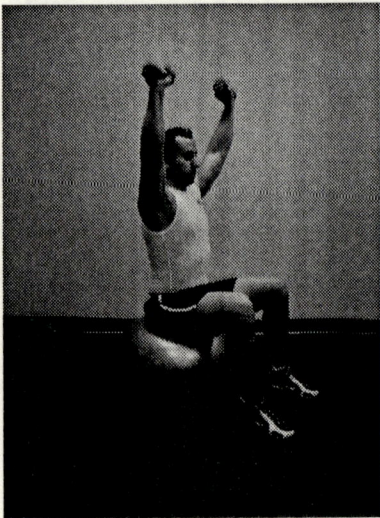

EXERCISE 3- **STEP-UPS**
Target area- Legs, cardio.

- PERFORMED THE SAME AS IN PREVIOUS WORKOUT.

EXERCISE 4- **ABS.**
Target area- abdominals

BEGINNER: Start
Lye flat on the floor with the knees bent and feet flat. Cross arms in front of you.

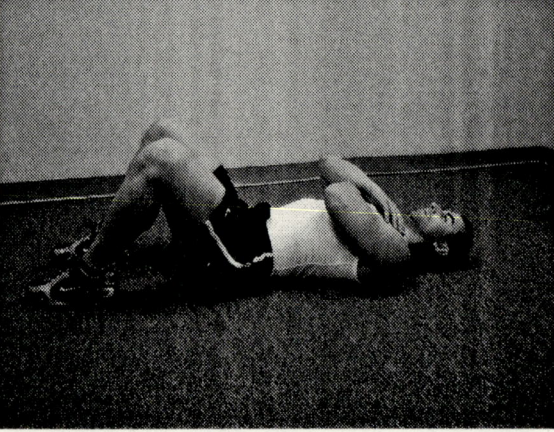

Finish:
Lift elbows up toward ceiling so shoulders lift slightly off the floor.

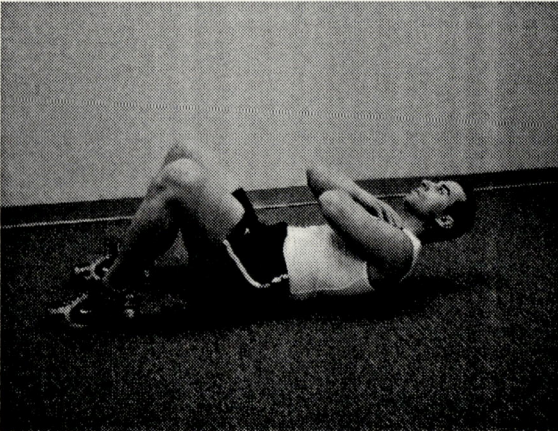

ADVANCED: Start
Lye flat on physioball with arms crossed in front of you.

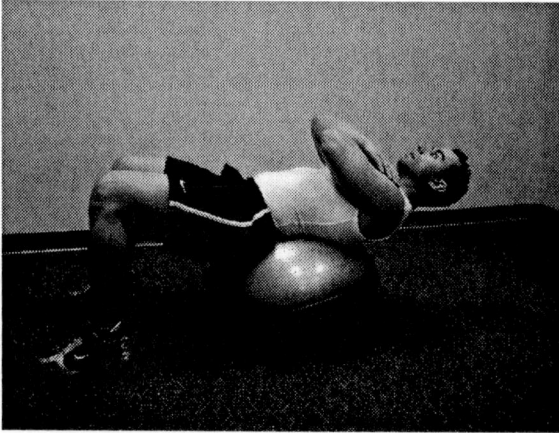

Finish:
While balancing on the physioball, lift elbows up toward ceiling.

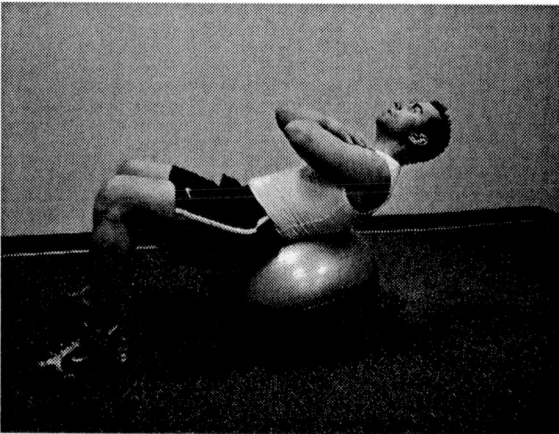

PROGRAM 2 (WORKOUT)
(Squats, Shoulder Press, Step-Ups, Abs.)
Weeks 1 and 2

PRESTRETCH

CHAIR SQUATS- (20 sec. on, 20 off)
SHOULDER PRESS- (20 on, 20 off)
STEP-UPS- (20 on, 20 off)
ABS.- (20 on, 20 off)
Complete 4x total

2-MINUTE REST

CHAIR SQUATS- (20 on, 20 off)
SHOULDER PRESS- (20 on, 20 off)
STEP-UPS- (20 on, 20 off)
ABS.- (20 on, 20 off)
Complete 4x again

POSTSTRETCH

PROGRAM 3 (REVIEW)
(Squats, Rows, Fly's, Lunges)

EXERCISE 1- **PLEAY SQUATS**
Target area- Legs

BEGINNER: Start
Begin by placing feet slightly outside shoulders with toes pointed outward. Hold a 5-pound dumbbell between your legs.

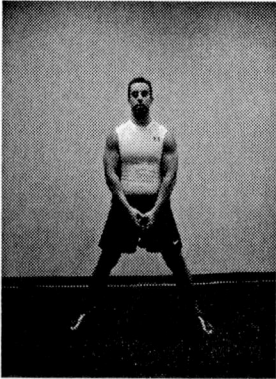

Finish:
Lower the butt half way down toward floor keeping the arms straight.

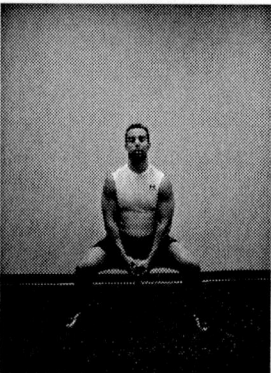

ADVANCED: Start

Begin by placing feet slightly outside shoulders with toes pointing outward. Hold a 5-pound dumbbell in between legs with arms straight.

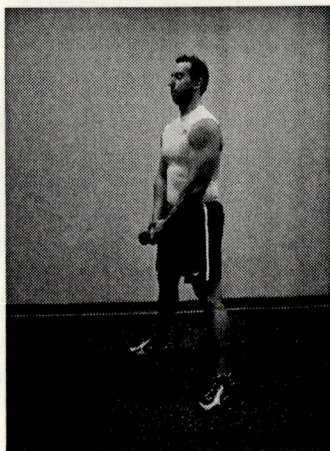

Finish:

Lower the butt half way down toward floor. As you lower the body, raise your arms so they are parallel to the ground.

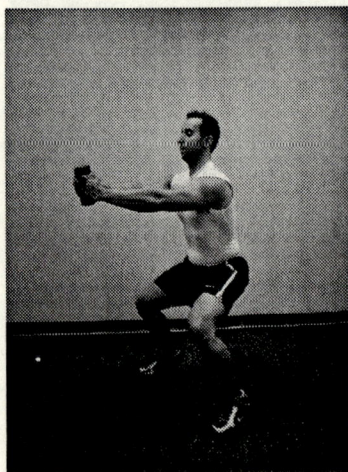

EXERCISE 2- **BENT OVER ROW**
Target area- back

BEGINNER: Start
Keep feet together with knees slightly flexed. Bend slightly forward keeping the back straight. Hold 5-pound dumbbells in each hand.

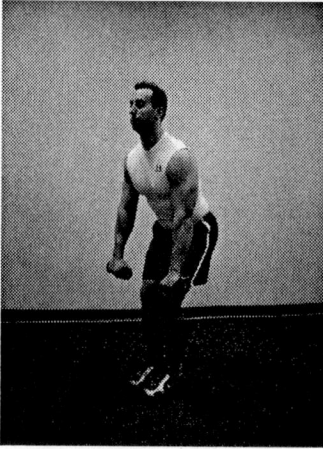

Finish:
Proceed to lift elbows toward ceiling.

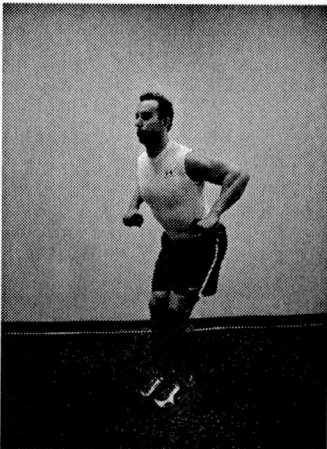

ADVANCED: Start
Keeping the body straight, place physioball underneath the stomach. Hold 5-pound dumbbells in each hand.

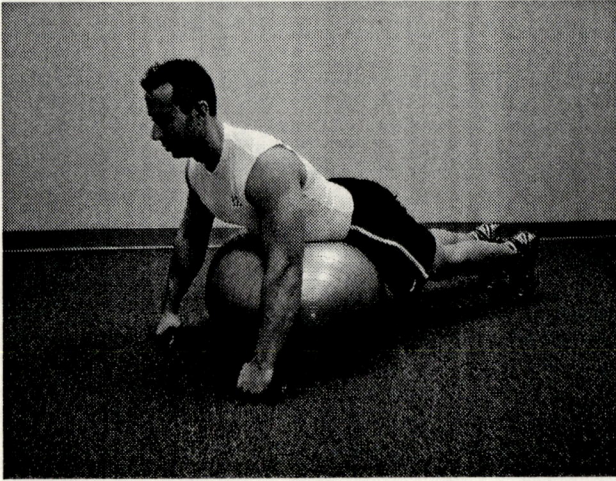

Finish:
Lift elbows toward ceiling.

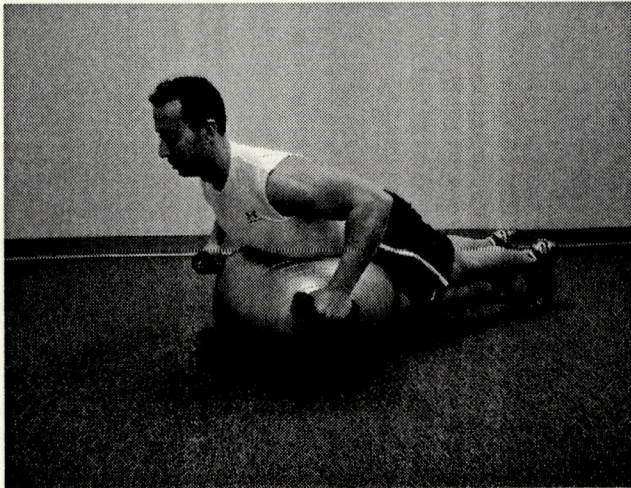

EXERCISE 3- **FLYES**
Target area- chest, shoulders

BEGINNER: Start
Stand with feet hip width apart. Hold 3-pound dumbbells
in each hand out to side with thumbs pointing upward.

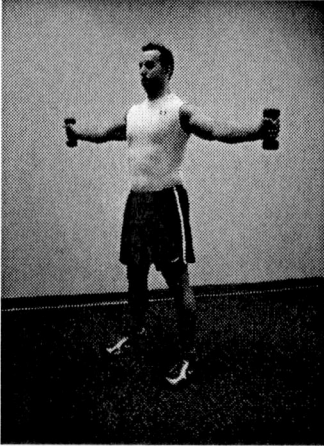

FINISH:
Bring arms together so they meet in the middle. Make
sure arms remain parallel to the ground.

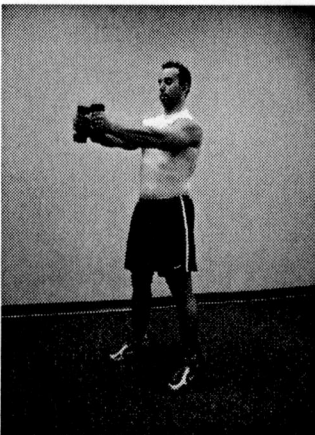

ADVANCE: Start

Lye flat on a physioball holding 5-pound dumbbells. Keep elbows slightly flexed.

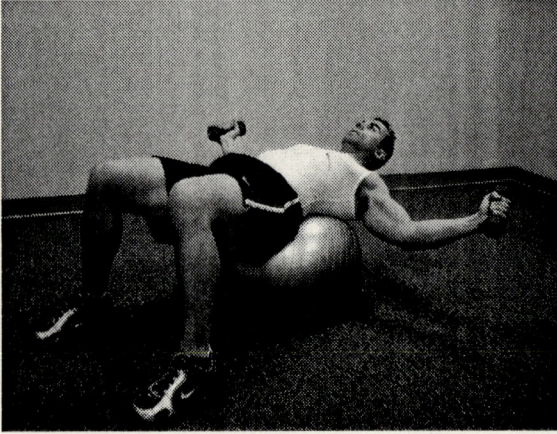

FINISH:

While balancing on ball, bring arms together so they meet in the middle.

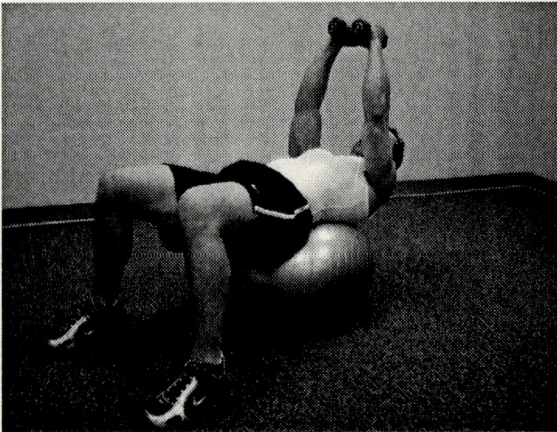

EXERCISE 4- **LUNGES**
Target area- legs

BEGINNER: Start
Hold onto railing or countertop with one arm for support. Keeping the back straight, place one leg in front of body and one in back of the body.

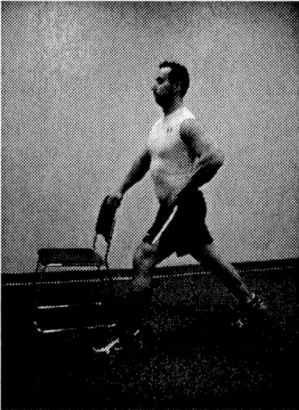

FINISH:
Lower butt toward the floor making sure the front knee does not travel past the front foot. If it does, create a larger space between feet.

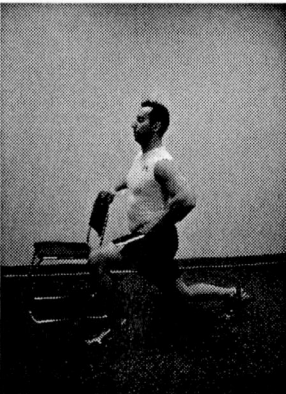

ADVANCED: Start

Hold 5-pound dumbbells in each hand. Keeping the back straight, place one leg in front of body and one in back of the body.

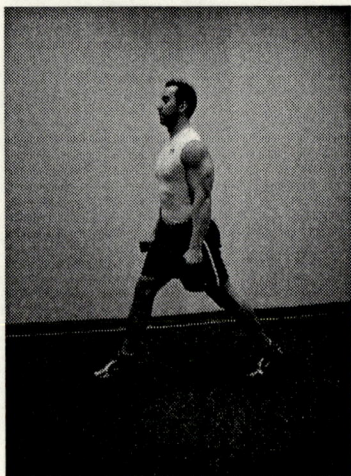

FINISH:

Lower butt toward the floor making sure the front knee does not travel past the front foot. If it does, create a larger space between feet.

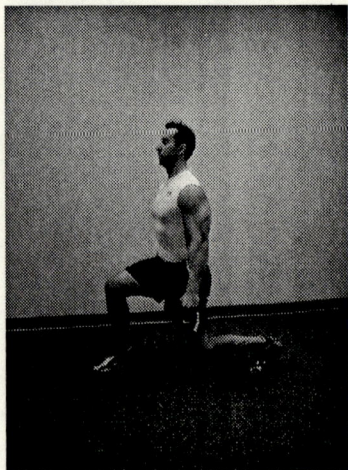

PROGRAM 3 (WORKOUT)
(Squats, Rows, Fly's, Lunges)
START AT WEEK 3

PRESTRETCH

PLEAY SQUATS- (20 sec. on, 20 off)
ROWS- (20 on, 20 off)
FLYES- (20 on, 20 off)
LUNGES- (20 on, 20 off)
* Complete 4x total*

2 MIN. REST

PLEAY SQUATS- (20 on, 20 off)
ROWS- (20 on, 20 off)
FLYES- (20 on, 20 off)
LUNGES- (20 on, 20 off)
* Complete 4x again*

POSTSTRETCH

PROGRAM 4 (REVIEW)
(Squats, Abs., Curls, Step-Ups)

EXERCISE 1- **SQUAT HOLDS**
Target area- Legs

BEGINNER: Start
Place physioball on lower back. Stand with feet hip width apart and forward. Keep hands on hips and back straight.

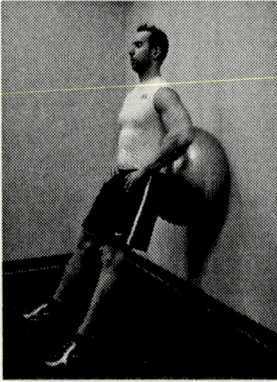

Finish:
Lower butt toward floor until legs are at a 90-degree angle and hold that position for 20 seconds.

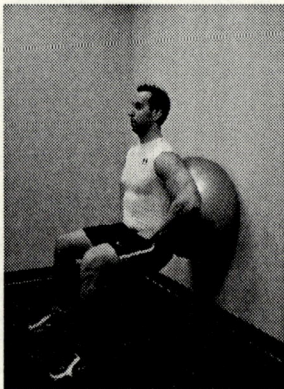

ADVANCED: Start

Place physioball on lower back. Stand with feet hip width apart and forward. Hold 5-pound dumbbells in each hand with back straight.

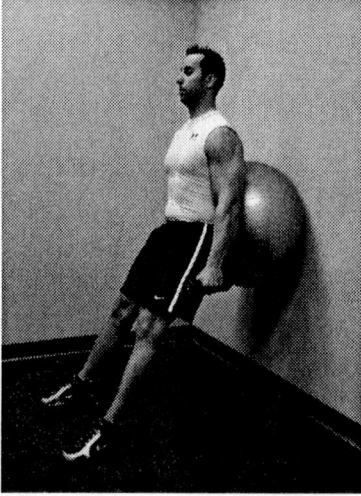

Finish:

Lower butt toward floor until legs are at a 90-degree angle and hold that position for 20 seconds.

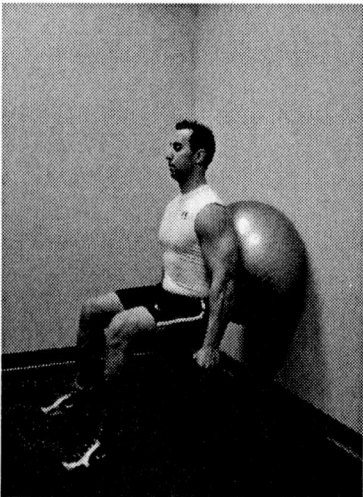

EXERCISE 2- **ABS.**
Target area- Abdominals

BEGINNER: Start
Lye flat on the floor with knees flexed and feet flat. Cross arms in front of body.

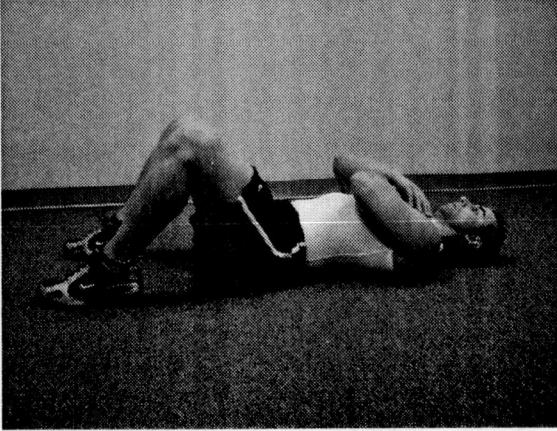

Finish:
Lift elbows toward ceiling. The shoulders should lift slightly off the ground.

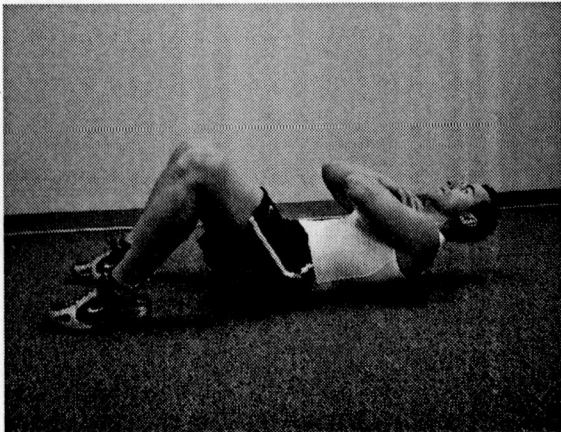

ADVANCED: Start
Lye flat on physioball. Cross arms in front of body.

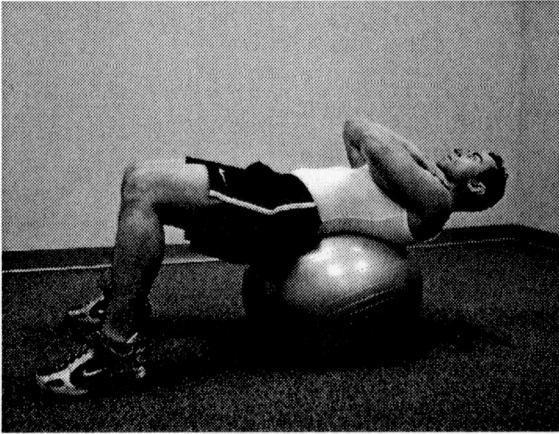

Finish:
Lift elbows toward ceiling. The shoulders should lift slightly of the ball.

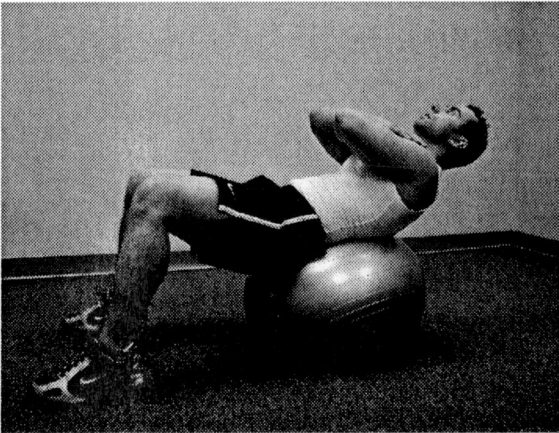

EXERCISE 3: **BICEP CURLS**
Target- Biceps

BEGINNER: Start
Stand with feet shoulder width apart. Hold 3-pound dumbbells in each hand.

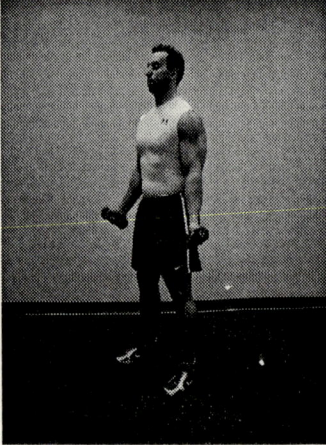

Finish:
Curl dumbbells upward. Palms of the hands should face up at end point.

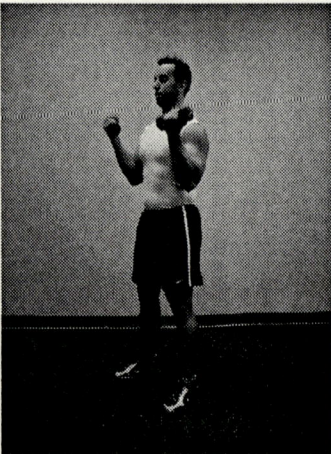

ADVANCED: Start

Sit on physioball with the back straight. Hold 5-pound dumbbells in each hand.

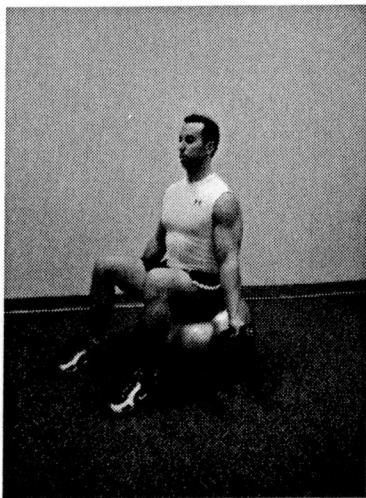

Finish:

Curl dumbbells upward. Palms of the hands should face up at end point.

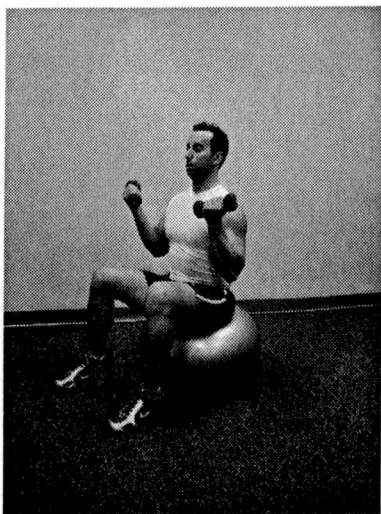

EXERCISE 4- **STEP-UPS**
Target area- Legs, cardio.

- PERFORMED THE SAME AS IN PREVIOUS WORKOUTS.

PROGRAM 4 (WORKOUT)
(Squats, Abs., Curls, Step-Ups)
START AT WEEK 5

PRESTRETCH

SQUAT HOLDS- (20 sec. on, 20 off)
ABS.- (20 on, 20 off)
BICEP CURLS- 920 on, 20 off)
STEP-UPS- (20 on, 20 off)
* Complete 4x total*

2-MINUTE REST

SQUAT HOLDS- (20 on, 20 off)
ABS.- (20 on, 20 off)
BICEP CURLS- (20 on, 20 off)
STEP-UPS- (20 on, 20 off)
* Complete 4x again*

POSTSTRETCH

APPENDIX I
GLYCEMIC INDEX OF COMMON FOODS*

Sugar	100
White Bread	100
Baked Potato	98
Carrot	92
Corn	82
Rice	82
Honey	75
All-Bran Cereal	74
Kidney Beans	71
Raisins	64
Pinto Beans	60
Yams	51
Oatmeal	49
Orange Juice	46
Rye Bread	42
Navy Beans	40
Apple	39
Yogurt	36
Skim Milk	32
Peach	29
Plum	25
Fructose	20
Soybeans	15
Peanuts	13

* From Springnet-Resource for healthcare Professionals

APPENDIX II
VITAMINS

1) <u>A</u>- Helps with vision, bone growth, healthy skin; acts as an antibody. (sweet potato, apricots, carrots, eggs)

2) <u>B1</u>- growth and development; aids in releasing energy from carbs. and protein. (spinach, beef, pork, nuts)

3) <u>B2</u>- digestion of fats; allows energy to be released from carbs. (cottage cheese, asparagus, meat, fish)

4) <u>B3</u>- helps to breakdown and produce glucose; maintains skin, intestines, stomach and nervous system. (red meat, poultry, kidney beans)

5) <u>B5</u>- aids in breaking down carbs., proteins and fats. (avocado, sweet potato, salmon, lentils)

6) <u>B6</u>- helps to digest and produce amino acids; aids in insulin production. (bananas, chicken, turkey)

7) <u>B12</u>- aids in nervous system function and processing fats and carbs.

8) <u>BIOTIN</u>- aids in carb., protein and fat conversion for body functions. (peanuts, cauliflower, spinach, cabbage)

9) <u>FOLATE</u>- helps to make DNA/RNA. (corn, chick peas, oranges, spinach)

10) <u>C</u>- Helps to form collagen; aids in tissue healing. (pineapple, strawberries, oranges)

11) <u>D</u>- Helps to form bones, teeth and cartilage by absorbing and using calcium. (egg yolk, salmon, tuna)

12) <u>E</u>- One of the most important antioxidant; prevents blood clotting. (almonds, peanuts, sunflower seeds)

13) <u>K</u>- Aids in blood clotting. (carrots, spinach, pears, grapes)

MINERALS

1) <u>CALCIUM</u>- found primarily in bones and teeth. (almonds, tofu, dairy)
2) <u>MAGNESIUM</u>- helps in muscle contraction; aids in bone and teeth formation. (red meat, legumes, nuts)
3) <u>PHOSPHORUS</u>- essential for bones and teeth. (dairy, seafood, whole grains)
4) <u>POTASSIUM</u>- helps to balance water in the body. (bananas, avocado, red meat)
5) <u>SODIUM</u>- controls amount of water in the body; helps with muscle contraction. (table salt)
6) <u>SULFUR</u>- helps to manufacture amino acids; converts carbs. to usable form. (dairy, chicken, seafood)
7) <u>CHROMIUM</u>- helps to bind insulin to its receptors. (apple, banana, grapes)
8) <u>COPPER</u>- production of hair and skin. (whole grains, sesame seeds, nuts)
9) <u>FLOURIDE</u> – increases bone density in teeth; decreases tooth decay. (teeth, bones)
10) <u>IODINE</u>- aids in metabolism and growth. (seafood)
11) <u>IRON</u>- helps in transporting oxygen throughout the body. (egg yolks, poultry, tuna)
12) <u>SELENIUM</u>- acts as an antioxidant; helps with immune system function. (shellfish, brown rice, poultry)
13) <u>ZINC</u>- helps to breakdown carbs., proteins and fats. (red meat, poultry, oat bran)

ABOUT THE AUTHOR

Kory Angelin received his degree in Sports Medicine and Athletic Training from the University of Charleston, and is also a Certified Fitness Instructor and Specialist in Performance Nutrition. Kory has worked in the fitness industry for the past 12 years and is President of FAST-EDGE Sports Performance. FAST-EDGE is one of the leaders in speed and conditioning for athletes. Their clients include numerous high schools, colleges and professional athletes. He received the "Above The Call Award" in 2002 from "Training and Conditioning Magazine" for his work in the health field and has been quoted in print in "Maxim Magazine". Kory has also been an on-air fitness expert for television in the local NY area, as well as, a guest speaker throughout the country. This is his first book.

Printed in the United Kingdom
by Lightning Source UK Ltd.
107232UKS00001B/224